Guide for House
and Interns
in the Surgical |

Eighth Edition

G. J. FRAENKEL

AM, MA, BM, MCh, Hon MD, FRCS, FRACS, FRACMA,
Hon FFARACS
*Coordinator of Research, Royal Children's Hospital, Melbourne.
Emeritus Professor and Foundation Dean, School of Medicine, Flinders
University, of South Australia. Former Ralph Barnett Professor of
Surgery, University of Otago, Dunedin, New Zealand. Former Surgical
Tutor, Radcliffe Infirmary, Oxford*

H. A. F. DUDLEY

ChM, FRCS (Ed), FRACS, FRCS
*Professor of Surgery, St. Mary's Hospital Medical School. Former
Foundation Professor of Surgery, Monash University, Melbourne,
Australia. Former Senior Lecturer, Aberdeen University, Scotland*

J. LUDBROOK

BMedSc, MD, ChM, DSc, FRCS, FRACS
*Associate Director and NH and MRC Senior Principal Research Fellow,
Baker Medical Research Institute, Melbourne, Australia. Former Dorothy
Mortlock Professor of Surgery, University of Adelaide. Former Professor
of Surgery, University of New South Wales. Former Senior Lecturer in
Surgery, University of Otago, Dunedin, New Zealand*

with

G. L. HILL

MD, ChM, FRCS, FRACS, FACS
*Professor and Chairman, Department of Surgery, University of
Auckland, New Zealand. Former Reader in Surgery, University of
Leeds. Former Assistant Professor of Surgery, University of Texas
Medical School, Texas, USA*

V. R. MARSHALL

MD, FRACS
*Professor and Chairman, Department of Surgery, Flinders University, of
South Australia. Senior Director of Urology, Flinders Medical Centre*

HEINEMANN MEDICAL BOOKS
London

Heinemann Medical Books,
22 Bedford Square,
London WC1B 3HH

ISBN 0–433–10804-5

First published 1961
Second revised Edition 1962
Third Edition 1964
Fourth Edition 1968
Reprinted 1971
Fifth Edition 1974
Sixth Edition 1978
Seventh Edition 1982
Reprinted 1985, 1986
Eighth Edition 1988

British Library Cataloguing-in-Publication Data
Fraenkel, G.J.
    Guide for house surgeons and interns in the surgical units.
    —8th ed.
    1. Surgery
    I. Title   II. Dudley, Hugh   III. Ludbrook, J.
    617   RD31

    ISBN 0–433–10804–5

Typeset by Observer Typesetting, Accrington
and printed in Great Britain by
Redwood Burn Ltd., Trowbridge, Wilts.

Contents

Preface to the Eighth Edition

This guide has its origin in loose leaf folders of notes which were provided to help house surgeons—and perhaps as importantly those who were about to become house surgeons—on the Professorial Surgical Unit at the Dunedin Hospital, Dunedin, New Zealand. The fact that the notes frequently disappeared, plus other indications of a wider demand, resulted in the publication of the *Guide to House Surgeons in the Surgical Unit* by the University Bookshop Ltd., Dunedin in 1961 followed by a second and revised edition in 1962. Since then the work seems to have acquired a life of its own.

The demands of different clinicians vary considerably on a whole variety of matters which relate to their patients, showing that the practice of surgery has wide room for variation. Nevertheless, there is sufficient common ground in general surgery—and certain of its more specialised aspects—to justify a guide such as this one. Its aim is to standardise various aspects of the management of patients suffering from common surgical conditions. Even if the team with which the house surgeon is working has different ideas, our text gives a starting point and also what we think is good general advice. Whenever possible, an explanation of the reasons behind a particular routine are given.

Everywhere that we have had the good fortune to work we have found common threads running through the way surgical patients are looked after, however much the detailed 'house rules' may vary. It is this, and the fact that our little guide keeps disappearing from the booksellers' shelves, which has encouraged us to keep the volume going.

Words change their meaning and we must admit that the terms 'house surgeon' and 'houseman' have become anachronistic for at least two reasons: first 'intern' is gaining ground as a general international sobriquet; second 'houseman' carries a chauvinistic overtone. We have persisted with the use of it and the general pronoun 'he'. This is not to underestimate in any way those house-women who have, in both professional and social ways lightened our task and provided a disproportionate amount of the cement that holds good surgical teams together.

G. J. Fraenkel, Adelaide; H. A. F. Dudley, London;
J. Ludbrook, Melbourne; G. L. Hill, Auckland;
V. R. Marshall, Adelaide
1987

ACKNOWLEDGEMENTS

We are indebted to the following for advice and information, and in some cases for detailed help with the manuscript. They must not, of course, be blamed for any errors or infelicities that we have committed.

In Australia and New Zealand

Dr R. W. Beal, Red Cross Blood Transfusion Service, Adelaide	Blood transfusion
Mr Brian Buxton, Cardiothoracic Surgeon, Melbourne	Transthoracic surgery; cardiac arrest
Dr D. E. Caughey, Consultant Rheumatologist, Auckland Hospital	Gout
Dr R. B. Ellis-Pegler, Physician in Clinical Microbiology, Auckland Hospital	Antibiotics
Prof W. S. C. Hare, Department of Radiology, Royal Melbourne Hospital	Radiology and imaging
Dr J. A. Judson, Intensive Care Unit, Auckland Hospital	Severe trauma
Dr Brendan Kearney, Institute of Medical and Veterinary Science, Adelaide	Laboratory reference ranges
Prof P. J. McDonald Department of Clinical Microbiology, Flinders Medical Centre, Adelaide	Microbiology
Prof T. S. Reeve, Department of Surgery, Royal North Shore Hospital, Sydney	Thyroid and parathyroid surgery

Mr A. A. Gunn,   Abdominal pain;
Bangour General Hospital,   appendicitis
West Lothian,
Scotland
Mr A. Sim,   Parenteral therapy
Academic Surgical Unit,
St. Mary's Hospital,
London
Mr R. deL. Stanbridge,   Transthoracic surgery
Division of Surgery,
St. Mary's Hospital,
London

Prof D. J. C. Shearman, Department of Medicine, Royal Adelaide Hospital	Gastric function tests
Prof A. G. Wangel Department of Medicine, Queen Elizabeth Hospital, Adelaide	Tests of immune function; antigens and antibodies
Dr J. A. Whitworth, Department of Nephrology, Royal Melbourne Hospital	Urine testing; renal function; renal failure

In the United Kingdom

Mr M. Aldridge, Academic Surgical Unit, St. Mary's Hospital, London	Individual diseases
Dr N. Carver Academic Surgical Unit, St. Mary's Hospital, London	General
Dr C. Coulter, Department of Radiology and Oncology, St. Mary's Hospital, London	Cytotoxic agents
Dr H. Dodsworth, Department of Haematology, St. Mary's Hospital, London	Blood transfusion
Prof C. Easmon, Department of Microbiology, St. Mary's Hospital, London	Antibiotics
Dr R. Elkeles, Department of Medicine, St. Mary's Hospital, London	Diabetes

Chapter 1

Administration

THE HOUSEMAN'S ROLE

A houseman occupies a unique position in the team of those who are looking after surgical inpatients. His role is complex, yet he is ill-prepared for it by those theoretical aspects of his undergraduate examinations upon which his teachers have exhorted him to concentrate. At one and the same time he is expected to be an organiser (getting patients from place to place, arranging their investigation and treatment), a scribe (keeping records and filling in forms), a guide and counsellor (seeing relatives and talking at length to patients about their problems), a minor executive (undertaking practical procedures), and an unfailing source of information to his senior colleagues on all aspects of those under his care. The diversified job specification is a daunting one, but at the same time it is the fastest way of bringing the new doctor to clinical maturity. He will get there quicker if he understands that the hospital is a very complex organisation, the structure of which he must master if he is to use its potential for the care of his patients.

A hospital can be looked upon as a set of discrete areas, each under separate control, all ostensibly there for the good of the patient, but all functioning largely independently of each other. The connections between them are made by the communication of data about patients and the passage of those individuals who have roles in more than one place from area to area. Prominent as both a communicator and as a man who gyrates between operating theatre, ward, outpatients and special departments, is the houseman. His success will be directly proportional to his basic understanding of how to communicate, how to arrange for things to be done to (and for) his patients, and to his being obvious as an individual who is prepared to exert himself in seeing that communication is not impersonal. To achieve the one he must rapidly come to grips with the technical details of which forms to fill in, which days to choose for certain investigations, which individual to approach for a given purpose. In this he may be assisted by

1

whatever local manual is produced by the hospital in which he is working, but such manuals are far from commonplace and usually he must pick up his skills in this field entirely by word of mouth and from a brief introductory course that his hospital may provide. To acquire success in personal contact it is necessary to devote time and thought to the process; 5 minutes spent in taking an x-ray request slip down to the department with a courteous verbal expansion of the details that have been written down, and a similar time devoted to delivering the theatre list in person to the reputedly draconian theatre superintendent, pay dividends out of all proportion to the effort involved.

The houseman should also not forget the informal communication network which exists in every organisation and is a particular feature of hospitals. More can often be accomplished by knowing and being on good terms with secretaries, porters, orderlies, and administrators than by cultivating the more Olympian members of the medical profession. Paramedical and non-medical personnel make up the skeleton of function upon which the flesh of nursing and medicine is hung. Their very permanence gives them a knowledge and authority which can be most useful if properly exploited and very humiliating if it is used to make the houseman feel inferior. Their friendly advice should rarely, if ever, be neglected.

One of the hardest things to learn about a hospital is that it is a place of tension. There is tension in the ill patient; the tension among those who worry about making him well (and also about the views of others as to their competence); the tension of long hours and irregular sleep patterns; and last, and perhaps most regrettably, the stress of an organisation that is too hierarchically organised. Many of these things are changing, but it is well to remember that when there are inexplicable rows, unworthy assignment of blame, and seemingly irrational behaviour, the human situation described may be the cause. As the bottom man on the totem pole, the wise house surgeon will not only scorn delights and live laborious days, but also keep his head even if all about him others are losing theirs. If he is wise he will be quiet in his comments and neutral in his attitudes.

It is regarded as bad form these days to write too much about commitment. Nevertheless, for what amounts to only a relatively short period of a professional lifetime, the only good house officer is a committed house officer. The organisation he serves and from which he will emerge clinically confident and ready to tackle his life's work should, for the time he holds the job, come first. In our experience, no one so engaged looks back with regret though he may sometimes do so with anger at 'things ill done and done to others harm which once he took as exercise of virtue'. There are hard knocks aplenty in being a house officer, but a great deal of enjoyment as well.

RESPONSIBILITY

It is difficult to lay down a clear division of responsibility within a unit, but the following general principle applies: if you are worried about a patient or some unforeseen complication arises, examine the patient as fully as possible and then *tell* your immediate senior—it then becomes *his* concern, and *his* responsibility as to whether he should see the patient or not. Likewise *tell* whoever is responsible for the emergency surgery of all emergency admissions as soon as you have examined them. A particular problem which often gives rise to confusion is when a patient is transferred to a specialist unit—e.g. the intensive therapy unit—during his hospital stay. Such units usually have their own house staff and routines and expect you to let them take responsibility for writing orders, drugs and fluid balances. This makes it difficult for you to maintain continuity in your care. Though it adds to your work load you *must* keep abreast of what is going on because if you do not the patient may suffer from the other team's lack of knowledge of what you know. When responsibility is handed back you will be out of touch.

Last, let us set a question to all potential housemen. If you have just gone to bed at 2 a.m. after a hard day and the night nurse calls to say she is still worried about Mrs Brown, what is your answer? For those of us who believe in responsibility in medicine there can be only one—'I'll be up to see her within 5 minutes.'

SOME PRACTICAL POINTS

1. Keep a notebook and write *everything* down, crossing it off as you do it. Do not use the backs of envelopes.

2. Try to end your day by filling in any forms that will be required for tomorrow. More generally try to anticipate everything so that it is done before it is needed.

3. Think ahead all the time—who is going home, who is going to need social care, who might be requiring further surgery and when.

4. Always reflect before you act whether or not you should inform someone else—you usually should.

5. Make sure that your immediate associates know what to do and when you need to be informed.

6. Try to request investigations so that the results will converge on a decision making point—e.g. a unit round or a time when the next operation list is being planned.

ADMISSIONS

All patients must be seen at the earliest possible opportunity and notes written up forthwith. Construct an investigation plan for every patient (see Records, below). Some tests may have been carried out or ordered from the outpatients department for those who are being routinely admitted. Others may be suggested in the notes. The following are useful guides. *All* patients who are destined for major surgery should have the following investigations at least considered:

Weight and height
Ward urinalysis
Full haematological screen (blood count, examination of a film)
Biochemical screen (including electrolytes and blood urea) for abdominal surgery
Chest x-ray in patients over the age of 40 who have not had a chest x-ray in the last year and/or have respiratory symptoms.
All patients over the age of 40 who are to undergo major surgery should, if resources permit, have a standard ECG taken.

In some hospitals:

Nose and throat swabs
Sickle cell solubility test in black patients.

In any patient in whom respiratory problems exist or in whom thoracotomy is contemplated, obtain:

Sputum culture

Vital capacity and forced vital capacity in one second (FEV_1)
(before and after bronchodilators)
Arterial PO_2 and PCO_2

Remember that consultations with others may be required at, or shortly after, the time of admission and if days are not to be wasted these should be set up at once. This is particularly true of the need to look after the psychosocial side of the patient, who may be more worried about wages or family care than about his illness.

Later in this Guide there are details of differential diagnosis to consider, and further investigations to undertake, in specific surgical conditions or situations.

Patients who are admitted as a matter of *emergency* present special problems, dealt with under individual headings. However, they may have a past history of surgical or other treatment elsewhere. It is not adequate to accept their version of such an episode—wherever possible you must aim to obtain the information direct by using the telephone to contact the records office of the previous hospital or the general practitioner concerned.

RECORDS

Most doctors do not enjoy keeping records. Yet time and time again the usefulness of past information to current management can be clearly demonstrated. Surprisingly, in spite of all such examples, we are still far from agreeing what should be recorded and how. Most conventional hospital records are dry as dust, little used as a day-to-day method of handling the patient's course, and often deficient in the items of information posterity wants. It is little wonder that the houseman senses a lack of interest from his seniors in the whole matter of record keeping. How then are we to preserve the good and necessary features of records, and at the same time generate enthusiasm for their completion?

One answer to this question lies in the use of what it has become fashionable to call 'problem orientation'. The conventional information on history and physical examination is collected as before, but it is used merely as a matrix against which all those concerned attempt to define a list of problems which confront the patient. Management and the recording of progress is then conducted with reference to this list, adding or subtracting to and from it as occasion demands and as new problems appear or old ones become inactive. The value of this approach is that the record becomes a dynamic vehicle for communication and there is usually also a much clearer delineation of the exact way in which the patient should be handled.

Problem orientation must start with the house surgeon who makes the initial problem list but it cannot end there; he is not alone in the exercise. If he is to make a record work in this way he must insist, cajole, wheedle or inveigle others into putting down their thoughts in concrete terms. Similarly in the surgical setting, operation notes are not very useful unless they are preceded by an explanation of *why* surgery was undertaken and contain in their text the argument why a certain course of action was chosen. This is particularly the case if they are part of the means of communication with the patient's doctor outside hospital.

The future of problem orientation in medical records is not exactly clear. In the meantime it is recommended as the basic way a record should be kept and particularly how the progress notes should be arranged. A brief example is shown below. As with many things, this is just an ordering and rationalising of what already happens, but with the advantage of leaving a clearer account of what actually took place for those who may have to scan the record and draw conclusions about the patient, either in your absence or at some future date.

Postoperative progress Mr H. F.

Problem list

1. Partial gastrectomy for DU.
2. Preoperative chronic bronchitis
3. Anxiety state.

Day 1. 1. Bowel sounds absent. Duodenal stump drain 90 ml. Nil orally; for gastrografin swallow tomorrow to see if oral feeding can begin.
2. Some coarse rales at right base. Chest x-ray shows increased hilar density only, without evidence of collapse-consolidation. Continue preoperative physiotherapy. No indication for antibiotics at this time but repeat physical examination and x-ray tomorrow.
3. Reaction to operation less acute than expected.

Continue diazepam 2 mg IM for next 24 hours on same schedule as preoperatively (6 hourly).

Day 2. 1. Bowel sounds present. Gastrografin shows contrast in terminal ileum at one hour. Begin oral fluids.

2. Chest sounds less and x-ray *not* taken. *Note by physiotherapist*—he is doing well but his sputum remains thick and he is wheezy intermittently; would bronchodilators be helpful? Thanks, yes we will prescribe.

3. No change. Consider withdrawing diazepam tomorrow but remember that he may have difficulty in sleeping.

Indeed there is much to be said for a single record used by everyone. This example includes one excellent feature of the problem orientated record namely that it is not exclusive to the medical profession as records have tended to be in the past.

Discharge summaries serve two purposes: they inform the doctor; and they act as an aide-memoire when the patient returns to outpatients or is readmitted. To a certain extent these purposes are in conflict and many hospitals have a short discharge sheet for the first and a longer summary (often unfortunately written up much later) for the second.

The first should contain:

1. A method of reminding the doctor outside the hospital about his patient—usually the presenting complaint.

2. What was done:
   (a) salient and positive investigations
   (b) treatment including operation(s) and date(s).

3. Major complications and outcome.

4. Discharge status and destination.

5. Drugs on discharge and supply.

6. Subsequent management needed from outside doctor (e.g. suture removal).

7. Follow-up arrangements.

8. In some instances advice about return to work.

9. What the patient has been told.

WARD ROUTINE

Find out from the senior ward nurse what is the most convenient time for you to do your daily round with her or the duty nurse. Also, ask what are the meal times and any other periods when it will not be possible for the nursing staff to accompany you, unless it is an emergency. It is unreasonable to arrive on the ward to see a non-acutely ill patient in the middle of dinner and then be cross because no one pays any attention to you.

MAKING ROUNDS

At the bedside get into the best position so that the assembled

Not this

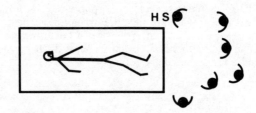

But this

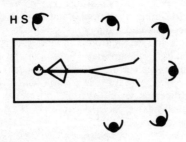

Figure 1

multitude can hear but the patient does not feel excluded (Figure 1).

Try to pitch your voice so that all involved can hear but in an open ward or multibedded bay not every other patient, porter or cleaner.

Avoid long dissertations.

Where possible use problem orientated expressions, e.g. 'This patient was admitted on Friday with a penetrating wound of the abdomen. Other significant findings were ...'. However, do not go beyond the facts—if all that is known is that the patient has abdominal pain or is jaundiced, say so.

Dry rounds. Some units like to have a discussion of the patient and his problems away from the bedside. There are advantages and disadvantages in this. The major advantages are: the patient is spared a long and incomprehensible discussion; the circumstances are usually better; all data can be marshalled and x-rays or other images examined properly; and, finally, use can be made of an overhead projector to summarise a case succinctly. The disadvantage is that facts on history and clinical examination are second hand (your hand). The onus is thus on you to have them as accurate as possible. It is essential that, if there is any doubt, the team goes to the bedside to re-check clinical facts. It is also vital that if conclusions about management are reached someone—often the houseman—must communicate them to the patient as soon as possible.

CONSULTATIONS

The transfer of responsibility or the request for advice is one of the most delicate matters in medicine. With increasing specialisation in the technology of care, there is all too often the tendency to call in an 'expert' who will deal with a part of the patient but not the whole. To avoid this unsatisfactory situation the request is usually made to a senior member of the unit to be consulted in the belief that he will concern himself overall with the patient. Each hospital has its own method of setting up this situation so that protocol is respected and propriety not offended. It is wise for housemen and registrars to undertake informal liaison at the same time as a more formal approach is being made; this permits some prior knowledge of what the consulted person is likely to expect in the way of attendance by a member of the team, special investigations, or arrangements for him to examine the patient in some particular way. Whether you transmit the formal request verbally (or, as is more usual and preferable, in writing) it is best, unless you are specifically instructed to the contrary, to make it a *request for an opinion*. In writing a request it should be in plain English, should avoid unnecessary details that can be obtained from the records, and should specify the problem for which the consultation has been requested. When more than an opinion is asked for, ascertain from one of the other and more senior members of your team what are the exact terms of reference—advice about some particular aspect of the patient, or to take over the management of the whole matter. When the matter is urgent by all means speak to the consultant concerned over the telephone, but it is a good thing to reflect whether such an approach might come better from someone else higher in the pecking order!

For ENT, eye and some other opinions where special equipment is needed it may be more convenient for the patient to attend the appropriate outpatient clinic.

RELATIVES

On all occasions you should be friendly and helpful to a patient's relatives. It is also important always to discover the precise degree of relationship, so that information is not given which might lead to subsequent difficulties. This situation occasionally arises with patients in whom for instance pregnancy or venereal disease is suspected or established.

With this proviso, it is one of your important duties to make sure that relatives are kept informed as to the nature of the diagnosis, likely operations, prognosis, or any deterioration in the patient's condition. When a patient's condition deteriorates unexpectedly, or a patient is to undergo an operation the outcome of which is uncertain, it is vital that a member of the unit informs the relatives in person or by telephone.

Close relatives who express a wish to do so are fully entitled to see the surgeon in charge of the case, and you may make an appointment for them to do so. You will find also that in some instances the surgeon himself will express a wish to see the relatives, and this is arranged as a rule to take place during or immediately after a ward round or outpatient session.

Difficulties may arise because the information given to patients and relatives by different members of the team either is, or appears to be, inconsistent. An active house surgeon will take the initiative as coordinator of what has been said.

THE REFERRING DOCTOR

It is important to remember that the patient's family doctor has entrusted the patient to your hospital unit for *specialised surgical care.* He will continue to be the physician and counsellor to the patient and his family when the former leaves hospital. At the very least, he must be informed within a very short time of the patient's discharge from hospital about the more important features of the *diagnosis, treatment,* and of *recommendations for further care.* If it is important that the patient consult him shortly after leaving hospital, both he and the patient should be informed. He must receive an accurate account of any *drugs* or other forms of treatment with which the patient should continue once he returns home. If a detailed written account of these matters cannot reach the family doctor within 48 hours, he should be given the necessary information by telephone or by a brief summary which accompanies or precedes the patient (see discharge summaries above).

If the patient should die in hospital, it is important that his family doctor be informed within a matter of hours: it may be to him that the family turns for information and advice.

THE PATIENT

It is an unusual person who is not disturbed by his admission to hospital. He may be more or less distressed by the unfamiliar and often *frightening environment,* by the uncertainties which surround an *operation,* by fears regarding his *physical ailment* and by anxieties in regard to his *domestic life or work.* The surgical resident plays a vital role in all these aspects of the patient's illness. Because of his frequent attendance on the patient he is often looked upon overtly or covertly by the patient as a counsellor. He fails in his duty if he does not spend the time that is necessary to explain the patient's illness to him, explain the circumstances which will surround his operation and the postoperative period, and recognise and attempt to alleviate any other source of distress to the patient.

The particular stresses to which surgical patients are exposed may sometimes lead to bizarre behaviour. Some patients become passive, apathetic and depressed; others aggressive and truculent; yet others excited and even occasionally disorientated. Normal traits such as obsessiveness may become exaggerated. Complete denial of the illness may occur. It is very important that the houseman recognises the possibility that the patient's behaviour is not normal, and that he takes this into consideration both in designing treatment (e.g. sedation) and in providing commonsense psychological counsel, (see also Acute postoperative mental disturbances, p.149). The reactions of patients to hospital admission are also culturally based. Care must be taken not to assume that what appears odd to you is necessarily abnormal to the patient.

Particular problems arise in patients who have cancer or are dying. In the past it has often been the custom to conceal the facts from the patient by the use of euphemism or tactics of denial which amount to untruth. As often as not this is misguided. In those who have firm faith of a religious kind, or who are well supported by close family ties or by friends, a conspiracy of silence can do more harm than good and frequently involves the medical staff and patient in contortions of evasion ultimately resulting in a loss of mutual confidence when, as it will, the truth comes out. The general axiom is that the truth, well put and hedged around with the appropriate and real uncertainties that must accompany any attempt to foretell death or disaster, should be the usual strategy. The exception is the lonely, self-supporting individual who has already shown strong denial mechanisms towards his illness.

The tactics used in bringing a patient to grips with a diagnosis such as cancer which is threatening to him, or with the finality of death, can only be cultivated by experience; clearly no doctor in his right senses bluntly and baldly puts the facts before his patient. As with other interviews it is best to encourage the patient to talk about his illness: sometimes it is clear from such preliminary skirmishing that denial is a strong force and no further action should be taken, nor has harm been done; sometimes it is immediately apparent that he knows or suspects and is anxious to talk the matter over. The recognition of the serious nature of the situation by the patient should lead the houseman to move on quickly to considering the positive side of the matter—how plans should be made and what physical and financial support can be arranged. Before talking to a patient about problems of cancer, death and disablement you should have discussed the matter not only with your medical seniors so that all are aware of the plan, but also with those who are going to help solve social and family problems. It is increasingly clear that the social worker is vital in the management of many situational crises of this kind and the houseman must learn from the outset how to work with her for the good of his patients. It is not enough to identify the possibility of a social problem, write a request for consultation by the social worker and then forget the matter in the hurly-burly of acute surgical action. The unique position of the houseman in relation to his patients gives him an understanding of facts and attitudes useful to the social worker and makes it necessary that he should be seen to be concerned as part of the team solving these problems. Again, cultural differences must be borne in mind. We all now live in a polyglot society and must understand our neighbours' differences as never before.

On the rare occasions when a patient asks directly if he has cancer or is dying, it is a legal obligation to give an answer which to the best of your belief is true. It is also important to give a clear explanation of diagnosis and prognosis to the patient's closest relatives, but it is not usually helpful, or indeed fair, to ask them to make the decision on what the patient should be told, however much you must draw them into the business of telling.

When it has been agreed to discuss matters of this kind with the patient or when he demands information, the facts and their outcome should always be recorded in the notes. Apart from being a basic part of the medical record, this avoids uncertainty for others in the future, especially when the patient returns and says 'doctor said it wasn't cancer' or 'nobody told me anything'. The team must also speak with one voice.

There are three problems which precede death. The first is a tendency of the surgical team to withdraw from the patient. Though wrong this is a natural expression of their frustration and sense of inadequacy. They see themselves as concerned with life not death. Junior staff who are most in contact with the patients must counter this escapist attitude and continue personally to support the dying patient. The same problem occurs *after* death. The team tends to move on, leaving the house officer to tidy up, talk to relatives, sign the death certificate and answer queries. In a good organisation some of these duties should be shared but this is not often the case.

A good house officer will involve others as much as possible but most of the work will fall to him.

The second is the presence in most hospitals of a cardiac arrest team. If they are to do their job effectively they must act rapidly and without debate. Thus they cannot easily pause to discriminate over the rights and wrongs of resuscitating an individual patient. It follows that the surgeons and nurses must, however distasteful it seems to be, discuss who should and who should not be resuscitated. In some institutions this also means writing in the record that a patient is or is not 'for resuscitation'. The important matter is that the house surgeon must be absolutely clear about how to proceed, even if he has to badger his seniors to get a definite answer.

The third matter is organ donation. The needs of the individual and the relatives must be balanced against the needs of others. No one wants to deny health and survival to the patient with chronic renal failure or irremediable cardiac disease. Equally, no one wants to confront the relatives of (say) a decerebrate patient with the imminence of death. However, the reality of life and death has to be faced. The houseman must be alert to the possibility of 'potential donors' and thus to put into action whatever local procedures exist. These will include certain approaches that have to be made to the relatives and the transplant team and baseline investigations on the patient. You should be sure about local arrangements so you are not caught unawares (see next section).

ORGAN TRANSPLANTATION

Not every hospital engages in organ allotransplantation, nor is the general surgical house surgeon necessarily involved. However, every hospital is a potential source of cadaveric donor kidneys and there has been an increasing use of hearts and livers for allotransplantation. Potential donor patients are aged between 10 and 50 years, with a lethal cerebral lesion, but with apparently normal renal, cardiac and liver function. Sepsis must be absent and patients with malignant disease are excluded. The need for all of these functions to be normal may not be necessary and will, to an extent, depend on the organ that is to be transplanted. The cause of the cerebral lesion will be head injury, spontaneous intracranial haemorrhage, cerebral anoxia from temporary cardiac arrest, or a brain tumour. It is becoming more common to remove organs before respiratory support is withdrawn, thus relying on brain death rather than the more customary diagnosis of death, namely, irreversible cessation of circulation or blood. The diagnosis of brain death was addressed by the Conference of the Royal Colleges and Faculties of the United Kingdom in 1976 (*British Medical Journal* 1976 **2** 1187-1188). In essence, brain death should be considered if:

1. The patient is deeply comatose and there is no indication that this is the result of depressant drugs, hypothermia, or metabolic and endocrine disturbances.

2. The patient needs ventilator support because spontaneous respiration is inadequate or absent.

3. The diagnosis of brain death is confirmed by demonstration that all brainstem reflexes are absent. The pupils should be fixed, there are no corneal or vestibulo-ocular reflexes, there is no motor response within the cranial nerves, the gag reflex is absent and no respiratory movements occur when the patient is disconnected from the mechanical ventilator.

Once the diagnosis of brain death has been made, permission needs to be obtained from the coroner, if appropriate, and from the nearest relatives before further consideration can be given to organ donation. In general, relatives should not be approached until it becomes obvious that death of the patient is inevitable. In most cases the hospital will have a definite policy on who is the most appropriate person to approach the relatives. This may be a member of the transplant team or a senior hospital doctor who may or may not have been involved in the management of the patient. The relatives' permission should be obtained whenever possible at personal interview and only on very rare occasions should it be necessary to discuss the matter by telephone. As a rule, a number of further investigations are made to determine the patient's suitability as a donor. Tissue typing, blood urea concentration, an intravenous urogram and an HIV antibody test are usually required before renal donation. The specific requirements will vary from unit to unit and will depend on the organ that is to be transplanted. Most transplant units or programmes have their own protocols and it is important to be aware of them so that the appropriate preparatory procedures can be undertaken. Perhaps the most important requirement is to notify the transplant units of a potential donor as soon as possible so that there is adequate time available for the necessary steps to be taken.

DEATHS

It is important that you notify all deaths to the immediate senior member of the staff responsible for the patient; at once in the case of unexpected death and as soon as is reasonable in predicted deaths.

Surgical units have sometimes been judged by the assiduity with which they seek and secure autopsies. This is admirable, but can be carried to ridiculous and painful lengths. A more enlightened attitude is to debate each instance on its merits, starting from the premise that reasons must be found for *not* having an autopsy. Autopsies are *your* direct responsibility, and if deaths occur when you are off duty, on your return you must check that permission has been sought. One should endeavour to ensure that a patient is not taken from the ward until all arrangements have been made.

In certain circumstances a death must be reported to the *coroner*. The rules vary in different parts of the world and even, for instance, between England and Scotland. In England and in many other countries: deaths in the operating theatre; deaths following (at whatever remove) accident or suspected crime; and unexpected deaths in a wide variety of circumstances must be reported. If certain words such as 'alcohol' appear on a death certificate, the death is automatically referred to the coroner. The coroner's office is almost always a helpful institution and a phone call is the best way of discussing any problem. You must consult if you are to avoid getting caught in a sandwich between your seniors and the coroner.

Always obtain the autopsy report.

OUTPATIENT FOLLOW-UP

In most units it is an invariable rule that every patient be seen at least once after his leaving hospital, in the outpatient clinic of the surgeon who carried out the operation or who was responsible for the investigation. This appointment should be for 2 to 3 weeks after leaving hospital, unless other instructions are given.

After one postoperative visit, many patients need not be seen again, and the patient and his family doctor should be informed of this. However, in most units patients with certain diseases will be followed up for very much longer periods. This is often true of patients with malignant disease; of patients with other diseases in which the unit is conducting a special study; or where for other reasons it is in the patient's interest to be seen regularly by a specialist surgeon.

PRESCRIBING

Prescribe precisely and you will benefit your patients, save money and stay out of trouble.

1. *Use the approved name*—the proprietary name may be added in parentheses. Some authorities now question this view because proprietary drugs vary in their potency and availability, but we continue to support it.

2. *Specify the dosage*—not just as '1 tablet t.d.s.' but as '0.5 g tablets 1 t.d.s.'

3. *Specify the route*—injections should be specified as IM or SC.

4. *Specify the duration of treatment*—whenever this is possible and always with antibiotics. On all patients check the prescription list every 24 hours and ask if particular drugs need to be continued. On complex problems insist on a 'therapy review' every 3 or 4 days, to be undertaken by all concerned.

MEDICINE AND THE LAW

In hospital practice the law interacts with medicine in three main areas: professional negligence, confidentiality, and certification. Both the law and its interpretation may differ substantially between one country and another, between state and state in countries where such devolution exists and may vary even from one city to another in the same state. In any case of doubt therefore you should always consult one of the administrative officers of the hospital, because in the majority of cases the hospital will also be involved in any medico-legal matter that is of concern to you.

The most important piece of advice *in regard to professional negligence* is that you should at all times carry the best insurance policy you can afford against claims for professional negligence, whether or not the hospital is also insured. The hospital's insurers will safeguard the interests of the hospital, which may conflict with your own. Many cases of alleged professional negligence are hard or impossible to defend because adequate records are not available. Let this be an additional incentive to you for keeping the fullest possible account. You should also spend one of your free evenings in reading the annual reports of some of the medical defence societies. They are often entertaining and instructive.

In regard to confidentiality there are certain easy guidelines. It is unwise to discuss a patient's case over the telephone and very much better to speak to the enquirer in person after it has been established that the patient wishes you to communicate the information, or that the enquirer is entitled to the information by virtue of a very close relationship. You must insist on having a signed consent form from the patient or his legal guardian before providing a written report about his medical condition to anyone except his personal medical attendants. All enquiries from the press about patients should be referred to the hospital administration.

In regard to certification read carefully any prescription or document which you sign and be sure that you hold all the qualifications necessary to sign such a document in that particular city. Be very sure to distinguish between fact and opinion, and never sign a document stating that you have carried out a certain examination or other procedure when in fact this is not the case. When there is any doubt whatever, consult an officer of the hospital or your medical defence society, or both. The matter of the certification of death presents great difficulties at any time, and never more so than when the issue of the donation of an organ for transplantation arises. The law and the practice of coroners and coroner's offices is so varied that it is essential for you to seek instruction as to the types of deaths of which the local coroner likes notification and the form in which he likes it. For instance, in some areas all cases of jaundice as the cause of death are automatically notified to the coroner because of past records of industrial poisoning in that town. You must study the preferences of the local coroner in regard to death certification, because in most countries a coroner has such very wide discretion that a coroner who dislikes the way you handle things can make your life very miserable indeed.

For how to handle some forensic problems see p. 230.

Chapter 2

Management of Operations

OPERATION LISTS

Nothing causes more difficulties than organising an operation list properly. The following factors are important:

1. Arrange 'clean' before 'dirty': in theory ventilation should make it possible for a 'dirty' patient to precede a 'clean' one but this is not usually safe. Patients with special risks (hepatitis B and HIV) must be indicated to the theatre team: local rules apply.

2. A patient for whom something outside the theatre is required (e.g. a frozen section or an operative cholegram) should be scheduled at a set time (usually the beginning of a list or after a first operation of highly predictable duration). This always helps smooth external relations.

3. It is a good idea to start with a small operation of fixed duration which allows a 'warm up' period and which gives the theatre staff a chance to set up for a longer and more complicated case at leisure.

4. If (1),(2) and (3) can be achieved, it is a good thing to give the more elderly surgeon—fixed in his ways and even sometimes quite busy—a chance to start at a set time.

The operation list that goes to the theatre should specify:
   (a) the procedure
   (b) the approach (e.g. transabdominal, transthoracic)
   (c) the position of the patient if it is to be unusual (e.g. Lloyd Davies)
   (d) any extras required (e.g. catheterisation)
   (e) extra procedures (e.g. radiology).

The house surgeon is advised to go through the check lists which follow for each patient before and after operation. Some of the items are then discussed in more detail.

PREOPERATIVE CHECK LIST

While the details of making the arrangements for a patient to be operated on vary from hospital to hospital, the house surgeon's responsibility is usually clear: to make sure that no essential steps in the process have been omitted. Most hospitals have a system, but most systems require the very active collaboration of the house surgeon.

The following is a list of items that the house surgeon should check for each patient who is to go to the operating room.

Has the *surgeon* been consulted about the patient or list of patients?

Has *theatre* been notified of the list, and does the list contain an accurate description of the intended *operation* and all that is needed for it?

Has the *patient* had both the operation and early postoperative course explained to him? Is it necessary or desirable to consult with his relatives?

Is a *stoma* contemplated? (See p. 210)

Has the formal *consent* form for operation been properly completed?

Are the *baseline* investigations in order and within normal limits?

Has the patient any *allergies* or *hypersensitivities*?
e.g.   antibiotics
        anaesthetics
        applications (e.g. iodine, adhesive plaster)

Is the patient on any *drugs* that should either be stopped or their route of administration changed?
e.g.   antihypertensives
        antidepressants
        anticoagulants

Does the patient require any new or additional *medication*?
e.g.   diabetic control
        antibiotics
        steroids

Has the *anaesthetist* been notified?

Do the *nursing staff* know which patients are to be operated on?

Special preoperative orders for patients:
    area to be *shaved*

    nasogastric tube? (see next section)
    IV infusion?
    urethral catheter?
  Any *special requirements* for the operation:
    blood cross match?
    peroperative *radiography*?
    frozen section histopathology?
    clinical *photography?*
  Any foreseeable *postoperative* requirements?
    intensive care accommodation
    physiotherapy

Preoperative Nasogastric Tubes

In **elective surgery** there is rarely a need for a preoperative tube. If one is thought likely to be needed either pre- or postoperatively it can be inserted on the operating table.

In **emergency surgery** it is often thought desirable to empty the stomach before anaesthesia is induced. However, bear in mind two things: semisolid food or clotted blood cannot pass through an oesophageal tube; attempts to pass a tube in a sick patient (particularly in shock) may initiate retching and vomiting which defeat the object of the exercise, and may even lead to aspiration into the respiratory tree. The conclusion is simple: do not pass a tube at all and cooperate personally with the anaesthetist in applying cricoid pressure.

Technique of cricoid pressure. The supine patient is asked to swallow and then to extend the head so that the oesophagus is stretched on the spine and is thus less likely to slip away when pressure is applied. The fingers then press back firmly on the cricoid cartilage as the anaesthetist induces anaesthesia and passes the endotracheal tube. Pressure must be unrelenting until the cuff is inflated and there is no doubt whatever that it is the trachea that has been intubated. Do not apply cricoid pressure if the patient is retching—oesophageal rupture may result.

PREOPERATIVE MEDICATION

General Anaesthetic

The anaesthetist should normally prescribe the premedication himself. If not, the following is a useful guide. Premedication should be given from $\frac{3}{4}$ to 1 hour prior to operation, usually by subcutaneous injection, but if there is any measure of peripheral vasoconstriction it *must* be given IM or IV.

Under 3/12	Atropine 0.2 mg
3/12 to 1 year	Atropine 0.3 mg
1 to 2 years	Atropine 0.4 mg
2 to 10 years	Atropine 0.6 mg
10 to 15 years	{ Morphine 8 mg Atropine 0.6 mg
15 to 60 years	{ Morphine 10 mg Atropine 0.6 mg
Over 60 years	{ Morphine 8-10 mg Atropine 0.6 mg

Morphine 10 mg approximately equals Omnopon 20 mg.

Local Anaesthetic

A suggested scheme is (but individual preferences vary widely):

	Triflupromazine	15 mg
	Pethidine	100 mg
Adult:	IM One hour preoperatively.	

Half this dose can be repeated IV immediately prior to operation if necessary, and further IV dosage may be used as required.

Child: Use a correspondingly smaller dose.

N.B.   Occasionally severe falls of blood pressure occur especially if the patient sits up.

IMMEDIATE POSTOPERATIVE CHECK LIST

Before you and the patient leave the operating theatre, a number of matters must be attended to:

Make sure that *biopsy* or *operation specimens* are properly packaged, (*e.g. histological material in the right fixative, bacteriological material in the right transport medium*), labelled, and accompanied by a request form

Make sure an *operation note* is completed (at least in summary, if it is to be typed in full later)

Check with surgeon and anaesthetist re *immediate postoperative instructions:*

pain relief
IV or oral intake
nursing observations required
management of tubes, drains, catheters
any special drugs, e.g. antibiotics
special care for individual procedures

GENERAL NOTES AND CHECKS ON POSTOPERATIVE MANAGEMENT

Daily Check List

Temperature, pulse, respiration: is there any untoward trend? If so why?

Fluid intake and output (urine and drains)?

Are orders (including fluid orders) up to date?

Have the appropriate tests been ordered for the next day (always complete forms the evening before at the latest)?

Can the patient take drugs by mouth that are at present being given parenterally?

Should antibiotics be stopped?

Are sutures ready for removal? In general:

(a) clips are removed from the neck on day 2 and from other sites on days 5–7

(b) sutures are removed from the neck and face on day 2 and from the abdomen on days 7-10

Is/are drain(s) ready for removal? In general drains that have been inserted for:

blood, are left 36-48 hours
chest drainage after thoracotomy, are left until a chest x-ray confirms full expansion, and drainage is less than 100 ml/day
suture lines are left for 5-7 days
pus are left until there is no further drainage and/or a sinogram fails to show a residual cavity

A tube inserted percutaneously into the gastrointestinal tract (gastrostomy, jejunostomy, T-tube drainage of the biliary tree) should be left for a minimum of 8 days—i.e. until it is unequivocally sealed off from the peritoneal cavity.

Biochemical management. Serum electrolyte concentrations after operation, while useful as a check on normality, are no certain method of ensuring that all is well. They tend to be carried out daily but unless the situation is changing rapidly, every second day is quite adequate. Once parenteral therapy has been stopped there is rarely any need to make further measurements unless the clinical context suggests something amiss. Urine electrolyte levels, combined with a knowledge of urine volume, are very useful in checking balance and are not done often enough. They are essential in assessing repletion of a potassium-deficient patient.

Haemoglobin should be checked on the third postoperative day in any patient who has had major blood loss at the time of accident or operation, and twice weekly in patients with sepsis or making a complicated postoperative recovery.

Suspicion of sepsis (see Temperature charts on p. 140). Examine the wound for tenderness, redness or discharge. Culture every available secretion. Take a blood culture and repeat until two consecutive cultures are negative. Have a blood film examined at the earliest possible opportunity for the presence of Doehle bodies. Consult on the appropriate antibiotic regimen and other investigations (see also patients on long term parenteral nutrition p. 95).

Patients on intravenous therapy. Check the IV site of all patients daily. Tenderness at the infusion point is an indication to change it. With or without this, intravenous infusions should ideally not run for more than 24 hours at one site.

Patients with indwelling catheters should have a urine culture taken every third day.

Removing drains and other minor procedures on the postoperative patient (see also p. 23). When a drain is to be removed or an *open* wound dressed without an anaesthetic, it should be a therapeutic premise to give the indicated dose of morphine sulphate by IM injection 15 minutes (or by IV injection 5 minutes) before the procedure. There may be exceptions to this rule if the patient is already sedated, or there is some other contraindication to the drug, but it greatly reduces the pain and discomfort of what doctors are too often prepared to regard as a 'minor' procedure.

Therapy check. For most patients the above rules and checks should suffice. For the *seriously ill* it is good practice twice a week to undertake a routine 'therapy check' at which all items of treatment are reviewed.

POSTOPERATIVE MEDICATION FOR PAIN RELIEF AND SLEEP

Much can be done by counselling the patient upon what is to be expected. The house surgeon should keep his techniques simple. Some general points are:

For minor surgery *one* postoperative administration of an opiate is adequate and can be followed by minor analgesics such as pentazocine 30 mg IM or aspirin.

For major surgery or in situations where pain is severe (e.g. occasionally after haemorrhoidectomy) an opiate should be prescribed in regular doses so that pain is abolished. It is no use writing '4 hourly p.r.n.' for in this circumstance the drug will only be given if the patient complains. The instruction should read '*strictly* 4 (or 6) hourly'. Usually this is only required for 24 hours and may, of course, need modification to suit individual circumstances.

The following dosages are a useful guide. (Children frequently do not require postoperative opiates, but if necessary it is safe to give morphine in the dosages recommended.)

It is good practice to use continuous infusions of opiates to control initial severe postoperative pain. A motor driven syringe is best for this purpose and usually a rate of 2 mg morphine an hour suffices. When the patient has recovered from the general effects of anaesthesia and is beginning to experience pain, 15 mg of morphine sulphate are drawn up in 5-10 ml saline and administered at the rate of 1 ml every 15–30 seconds until pain is

Under 10 years	Morphine 0.2 mg/kg up to 4 hourly
10 to 15 years	Morphine 8-10 mg up to 4 hourly
15 to 60 years	Morphine 10 mg
or	Omnopon 20 mg
or	Pethidine 100 mg up to 4 hourly
Over 60 years	Morphine 8-10 mg
or	Pethidine 50-100 mg up to 4 hourly

completely relieved and, in the case of an abdominal or thoracic operation, respiratory movements are completely free. This 'titration dose' is then used to determine the rate of delivery on the basis that the dose, divided by 6, is the hourly rate. If opiate drugs have been used for the anaesthetic and particularly if opiate reversal with naloroxone has been undertaken, great caution should be observed with this technique.

Other methods of pain relief are gaining popularity, particularly extradural administration of morphine or other opiates. You should be clear exactly what is to be done and by whom, and where to turn for advice.

In the relief of acute pain of known origin preoperatively, insufficient use is made of the same technique of taking 15 mg of morphine, diluted in 10 ml of saline and injecting this intravenously at a rate of 1 ml/30 s until pain is relieved. Not only is this a very quick way of obtaining relief, but also a small total dose, 5-7 mg, is usually required.

The use of continuous intravenous morphine does carry a slight risk of overdosage characterised by a drowsy uncooperative patient, sometimes with a slow respiratory rate. This situation then joins the host of others that are responsible for mental confusion in the postoperative state (see p.149). The diagnosis can be made and the situation reversed by the use of naloxone hydrochloride 400 μg intravenously, repeatedly if necessary. The patient will recover but the postoperative pain for which the morphine was given will also recur.

Do not forget that the patient needs sleep as well as relief from pain. Sleep rhythms are disturbed after surgery and help is often needed, particularly when the patient is trying to convalesce in an open ward. The methods of providing sleep in the postoperative patient seem to change almost by the year. Barbiturates are rather out of fashion for this purpose but if they are habitually being taken they are better continued. For the anxious patient, injectable diazepam 2-5 mg is sound. For those who can take drugs by mouth nitrazepam (5-10 mg) is usually satisfactory. Avoid ringing the changes on these or any other drugs of common properties such as antidepressants. The differences are usually small and their therapeutic efficacy is at least in part based on your understanding of the circumstances and your 'feel' of how they should be used. The latter can only be acquired if you stay with a small number of preparations.

MINOR PROCEDURES UNDER LOCAL ANAESTHESIA

The houseman will often be called upon to undertake minor procedures, including supervising ward dressings. There is a natural tendency to be a little callous about these, but a little local infiltration for even the most trivial procedure will earn you the patient's thanks.

This Guide is not a textbook on techniques and you must look elsewhere, particularly to your immediate seniors, for firm guidance. However, the following general points are applicable:

1. Always use adequate preliminary sedation. Insert a butterfly needle. Give a small dose of morphine sulphate (5-10 mg) intravenously plus a little chlorpromazine (5-25 mg). This detaches the patient from his environment and so makes you and him feel more at ease.

2. Infiltrate *widely* with dilute local anaesthetic.

Lignocaine is the standard anaesthetic.

    (a) *The maximum* 'safe' dose of this drug is about 0.5 g

$$= \ 100 \ ml \ 0.5\% \ solution$$
$$= \ 25 \ ml \ 2\% \ solution$$

The 0.5 % solution should be used for all common purposes other than special nerve blocks.

(b) When *adrenaline* is included with the lignocaine solution, the concentration is such that the maximum 'safe' dose of adrenaline (0.5 ml 1/1000) will not be exceeded unless that of lignocaine is also. Adrenaline should *never* be used in a digital nerve block. Adrenaline should be used with caution in patients with some forms of heart disease.

(c) If *overdosage* of lignocaine should occur (muscle twitching, convulsions):

ensure airway, by intubation if necessary

give oxygen

give thiopentone IV slowly till convulsions cease

call an anaesthetist.

3. For lymph node biopsy make an adequate incision (4 cm) so that you are not struggling for exposure or to control bleeding. If you make a good job of suture the scar will be invisible. Don't pull on the node—the pathologist will hate you!

4. For needle cutting biopsies such as breast, liver or prostate make sure:

(a) you understand the way the needle cutting combination works

(b) you have incised the skin with a pointed scalpel

(c) you are aware of the hazards (e.g. the need to keep the patient still during liver biopsy)

(d) you have learnt the 'house rules' for the procedure.

5. If the lesion for biopsy appears to you to be doubtful (e.g. a possible malignant melanoma) don't do it—seek advice.

6. Don't hesitate to request technical help. Procedures may be thrown at you because you are thought to be competent. You lose nothing by admitting inexperience.

Chapter 3

Medical Factors in Relation to Surgical Procedures

DIABETES MELLITUS

Newly discovered diabetes mellitus should be adequately treated before elective surgery is undertaken.

Management During Surgery

Objective

1. To achieve good diabetic control postoperatively and especially to avoid ketoacidosis.

2. To avoid hypoglycaemia during anaesthesia. Consultation should take place between anaesthetist and clinician whenever possible.

The following should also be remembered:

(a) Blood glucose can be satisfactorily monitored on the ward using commercially available reagent strips without the necessity for a machine (e.g. BM strips or Visidex). Blood glucose can also be measured with the aid of monitoring machines with the appropriate strips. It is of utmost importance to ensure that all—nurses and junior doctors—are trained in their use, otherwise misleading results will be obtained.

(b) A satisfactory level for blood glucose control is between 6 and 12 mmol/l. This level steers a course between hypoglycaemia and hyperglycaemia.

(c) Anaesthesia and surgery will usually cause a rise in blood glucose as a result of the metabolic response to trauma.

(d) Insulin can be given parenterally both by addition of insulin to infusion bags, e.g. 5 or 10% dextrose given as a continuous infusion, or with the use of small volume infusion pumps. The advantage of adding insulin to dextrose is that insulin and dextrose are given together thus avoiding the potential problems of hypoglycaemia or mechanical failure of the pump. The disadvantage is that to change the amount of insulin involves changing the infusion bag.

Patients Who are on Dietary Management Alone

For minor operations no special precautions are necessary. For major operations, avoid glucose–containing solutions during the operation if possible. Postoperatively, monitor blood glucose carefully 4–6 hourly. Soluble insulin or equivalent may be necessary to control blood glucose given either b.d. or t.d.s. subcutaneously, or by addition to the infusion bag.

Patients on Oral Hypoglycaemic Agents

For minor operations no special precautions are required. In patients taking chlorpropamide, check blood glucose preoperatively to ensure that the patient is not hypoglycaemic because of the long half–life of this drug. For major operations, if the patient is well controlled, leave on current treatment. If the patient is taking chlorpropamide, replace this where possible 48 hours preoperatively with a shorter acting drug. Otherwise, check blood glucose preoperatively to ensure that the patient is not hypoglycaemic. If patients are poorly controlled they should be transferred to a twice daily insulin regimen preoperatively. During operations, blood glucose can be controlled with a dextrose/insulin infusion; usually between 1 and 3 units/hour are required. Postoperatively blood glucose should be monitored 4 to 6 hourly. The amount of insulin given can be varied to keep blood glucose in the acceptable range.

Patients on Insulin

Not all patients taking insulin are truly insulin dependent. Some have been treated with insulin because oral agents have failed while others are completely deficient in endogenous insulin production and will become ketotic if deprived of insulin even for short periods. Unless details of the history are known, it is safest to assume that all diabetics on insulin are insulin dependent. For very short operations, e.g. dental procedures, it is possible to omit insulin until the patient is able to take fluid and food by mouth a few hours later and then to restart subcutaneous insulin. For all other operations dextrose and insulin should be given intravenously. The amount of insulin required can be judged from the patient's normal daily insulin requirement. Usually 1 to 3 units/hour is sufficient. Postoperatively blood glucose should be monitored 4–6 hourly for at least 24 hours. When the patient can take food and fluid by mouth, change to subcutaneous insulin b.d. or t.d.s. A useful combination is soluble insulin before breakfast, soluble insulin before lunch, and soluble and isophane insulin before the evening meal.

Special Problems

1. *Emergency surgery*. Dextrose/insulin infusion should be used. Sepsis markedly increases insulin requirements.

2. *Cardiac surgery*. Patients undergoing cardiac bypass operations often receive large amounts of dextrose intravenously. This, together with hypothermia and inotropic drugs, may produce insulin resistance and drastically increase requirements for insulin.

CHRONIC RESPIRATORY DISEASE

This is common in those presenting for operation and most frequently is of the type broadly described as 'obstructive airways disease'. Often much can be done to improve respiratory function especially before a planned operation. Patients with respiratory disease should usually be admitted several days earlier for elective surgery.

Undertake respiratory function studies and baseline arterial blood gas in patients with:

1. Past history or present evidence of respiratory disease particularly chronic bronchitis or asthma.

2. Current cough or sputum or evidence that this occurs in unfavourable circumstances (e.g. winter).

3. Physical condition of the chest wall which may produce a restrictive defect.

In all these circumstances and in particular in the anticipation of major abdominal or thoracic surgery it is necessary to know three things:

1. Is the vital capacity (VC) greater than three times the tidal air?

If it is not, then respiratory insufficiency is almost inevitable after a laparotomy or thoracotomy, the muscular disorganisation and pain of which are sufficient to reduce VC by about two thirds. With appropriate action by the anaesthetist and the relief of pain (for example by epidural anaesthesia or continuous low dose intravenous morphine, p. 25) such patients need not go into respiratory failure, but this is only true if all are prepared by appropriate information.

2. Is there an element of bronchospasm? This can be ascertained by measuring forced expiratory volume (FEV_1), before and after the administration of bronchodilators such as an isoprenaline spray or a salbutamol inhaler. The presence of bronchospasm is an indication of likely postoperative trouble from sputum retention, and calls for postponement of the operation until control of the situation can be achieved.

3. Is there a restriction on free chest movement? A patient's FEV_1 may be low in the absence of airways obstruction if the lung and/or the chest wall are stiff. Such patients faced with additional burdens in the postoperative period may develop respiratory failure or, just as important, may get fatigued. Again appropriate avoiding action can be taken if the risk is understood.

In addition, when possible:

1. Choose the summer months for operation.
2. Stop patients smoking for at least 10 days.
3. Instigate active physiotherapy.
4. Give as early warning as possible to the anaesthetist.

HEART DISEASE

Previous myocardial infarction, or chronic angina of effort do not necessarily render planned surgery dangerous. Elective surgery is also safe following successful coronary artery bypass grafting. However, *recent* myocardial infarction adds greatly to the risks and elective surgery should not be done within 3 months and preferably not within 6 months of such an event. The risk is also high in patients with *unstable angina* and these should seldom, if ever, undergo elective surgery. Take special care of patients who require surgery as a consequence of recent myocardial infarction (retention of urine from diuretics; peripheral arterial embolus; peripheral arterial or deep venous thrombosis).

The risk of other forms of heart disease is usually proportional to the degree of exercise intolerance. However, beware also uncontrolled dysrhythmia and the stenotic mitral or aortic valvular lesion, especially when substantial blood loss may occur.

Any patient with clear–cut bradycardia should be referred to a cardiologist for an opinion as to perioperative pacing.

Antibiotic cover is essential for patients with heart valve disease or with a prosthetic valve undergoing any procedure, however minor.

For cardiac patients on anticoagulants see p. 36.

HYPERTENSION

1. Hypertension per se in the absence of cardiac failure gives rise to few difficulties during or after operation, provided any treatment which the patient normally receives is maintained.

2. It is most important that the anaesthetist is made fully aware in good time of any and all treatment for hypertension.

3. With modern drugs more problems arise from the withdrawal or modification of treatment than from continuing the normal regimen.

4. Nevertheless, the patient on antihypertensive treatment is likely to have lost normal haemodynamic reflexes. Therefore, very accurate fluid balance to avoid depletion or overload is essential.

CHRONIC RENAL FAILURE

Despite their metabolic disturbance and chronic anaemia, patients with renal failure tolerate surgery surprisingly well.

1. Plasma creatinine, urea and electrolytes should be measured before and immediately after operation. Urine should be cultured preoperatively.

2. If the cause of the chronic renal failure has not been established, medical referral is indicated.

3. The patient with chronic renal failure excretes relatively fixed amounts of sodium and water, and usually requires perioperative water and sodium infusion to maintain hydration and preserve renal function. Dextrose solution is best avoided as inability to excrete a water load can lead to dilutional hyponatraemia and a propensity to cardiac arrhythmia. Maintenance of a good urine output during operation minimizes the risk of superadded acute renal

failure.

4. Blood transfusion fails to correct the anaemia of chronic renal failure, and may further impair renal function. It should be reserved for replacement of blood loss.

5. Preoperative anaesthetic consultation is essential in view of problems such as acid–base status, fluid balance, and hypertension. In addition, renal failure alters the pharmacokinetics of certain drugs (e.g. sodium thiopentone), suxamethonium causes hyperkalaemia, and *d*-tubocurarine or gallamine can cause prolonged paralysis.

PATIENTS ON ADRENOCORTICAL STEROIDS OR ACTH THERAPY

These are used in a wide variety of conditions, e.g. rheumatoid arthritis, ulcerative colitis, 'collagen' disorders, anaemias, liver disease, asthma. Their significance with respect to surgery is:

1. They may *precipitate* a surgical emergency or mask its onset, e.g. perforation or bleeding from a peptic ulcer.

2. Under conditions of stress such as *operation* the normal pituitary–adrenal response may be so suppressed that relative adrenal insufficiency exists with the production of dramatic *arterial hypotension*.

The tests for pituitary–adrenal suppression are too elaborate for routine use. Thus it is *vital* to any person receiving, or who has recently received (within the past year) these drugs that added systemic corticoids be given over the period of operation. Such therapy should include consideration of those who have been on topical therapy (e.g. prednisolone enemas for ulcerative colitis).

Replacement therapy may also be necessary in operations directly on the adrenal glands. Finally, and uncommonly, therapeutic use of steroids may be required in unexplained hypotension where there is a possibility that 'adrenal apoplexy' has occurred—meningococcal septicaemia and head injury. These circumstances are rare. Apart from these uses the 'blind' administration of massive doses of steroids has *not* been shown to have any therapeutic influence on the course of inhaled vomit (Mendelsohn's syndrome); acute pulmonary oedema of other cause; adult respiratory distress syndrome; acute (as distinct from chronic) brain oedema. In spite of these negative findings, steroids are often prescribed in these conditions and may have deleterious influences on wound healing and erosive upper gastrointestinal lesions.

Replacement and Supplementation

1. The oral route should not be used during the perioperative period.

2. Intravenous agents act immediately and IM quickly.

3. 5 mg prednisolone or prednisone is equivalent to 25 mg cortisol (hydrocortisone).

Dosage Schedule (as hydrocortisone):

Evening before operation	100 mg IM
Day of operation	100 mg IM b.d.
plus, during operation	100–300 mg IV
First postoperative day	100 mg IM b.d.
Then 3 days	50 mg b.d.
3 days	25 mg b.d.

Then:

Replacement	**Supplement**
Start permanent maintenance dose of cortisone, 12.5 to 25 mg b.d.	3 days 12.5 mg b.d. then stop

plus fludrocortisone 0.1 mg daily.

Note: (a) If in either situation a postoperative complication such as infection should occur, it is important to maintain the dose of *at least* 100 mg daily till recovery.

(b) BP readings are probably the best early check on inadequate corticoid dosage. They should be made half-hourly for the first 48 hours and thereafter 4 to 6 hourly. If hypotension persists, estimate electrolytes in blood and correct any deficiency, especially low sodium concentration.

THERAPEUTIC STEROIDS

Therapy may be *local* or *systemic*.

Local

Hydrocortisone hemisuccinate 100 mg in 100 ml of saline or prednisolone 20 mg in 100 ml of saline or as disposable enema.

Given once or twice daily as a retention enema, the foot of the bed being elevated for 1 hour after administration.

Systemic

Prednisone or prednisolone, oral, IV or IM up to 40 mg daily.

PATIENTS ON LONG-TERM ANTICOAGULANTS

Many patients receive oral anticoagulants on a long–term or permanent basis, e.g. after heart valve replacement. The following are relevant for the houseman:

1. At the time the patient is encountered therapy may be
   (a) at the right level
   (b) non-existent
   (c) excessive.
Therefore the first thing is to check the prothrombin time.

2. Anticoagulant therapy may cause apparent acute surgical emergencies, e.g. bleeding into the wall of the distal small bowel or into the psoas muscle.

3. Patients well controlled on antiprothrombin drugs can undergo elective surgery without danger.

4. If anticoagulant therapy is mandatory but it is judged not wise to continue antiprothrombin drugs, continuous intravenous heparin should be used (p.144).

5. Reversal of the action of antiprothrombin drugs is by fresh frozen plasma (0.5–1 litre) and intramuscular Vitamin K (20 mg repeated 6 hourly).

JAUNDICE

Drugs, too numerous to list, can produce cholestatic jaundice that may mimic extrahepatic biliary obstruction. Postoperative jaundice may have a surgical or infective basis, and in minor degrees is a worrying associate of total parenteral nutrition, but may also occur from the use of halogenated hydrocarbon anaesthetic agents or at a later time from viral hepatitis. It nevertheless remains more common for the physician to manage patients with extrahepatic biliary tract obstruction medically, than it is for the surgeon to make the converse mistake.

GOUT

This is a common condition, particularly in males and is remarkably common in Polynesians. An acute attack (perhaps the first) may be precipitated by an injury, operation or illness such as myocardial infarction. Patients with established gout often know when they are developing an attack.

An acute attack is treated either with a non-steroidal anti-inflammatory drug, e.g. indomethacin 50-100 mg 6 hourly, with meals; or with colchicine 1 mg loading dose and 0.5 mg hourly until pain relief or diarrhoea occurs. If the patient cannot take drugs orally, indomethacin suppositories 100 mg are preferable to intravenous colchicine.

Allopurinol in a dose of about 300 mg daily is very effective in preventing recurrent acute attacks of gout. However, the initiation of allopurinol therapy may of itself precipitate an acute attack, so that there should be appropriate cover with indomethacin or colchicine.

Chapter 4

Laboratory Investigations

GENERAL

There are three good reasons and one bad for doing investigations. The good are:

1. To enable a *decision* about diagnosis or management to be made.
2. To *screen* individuals at risk for particular conditions which may affect their management.
3. To establish a *baseline* against which change can be studied.

Examples of the first are liver function tests and ultrasound examination in the diagnosis of jaundice and a serum amylase estimation in a patient who collapses with acute abdominal pain shortly after partial gastrectomy.

Examples of the second are chest x-rays before surgery and electrocardiographic studies in patients with degenerative peripheral arterial disease.

Examples of the third are serum electrolyte concentrations in patients undergoing gastrointestinal surgery and preoperative laryngoscopy in thyroid surgery.

The bad reason is because you were told to do it in case it was 'wanted' or 'might prove useful'.

House surgeons are not always free agents but they should carry this classification in their mind and resist the temptation to do what are often unpleasant and costly procedures unless they fit into the framework of management.

SOURCES OF ERROR

Although the results of these investigations are reported numerically, they are not necessarily more accurate than clinical findings in an individual case. That is, laboratory findings are subject to error.

38

The chief sources of error are:

1. *Sampling errors.* These apply to the collection of all specimens, and the source of error may be quite obscure unless specifically sought. So far as blood sampling is concerned, certain elementary precautions must be taken:

(a) *surgical spirit* (70%) only should be used as skin preparation. Small amounts of detergent entering the sample via the needle may result in significant haemolysis

(b) use a sterile, plastic, *disposable syringe and a disposable needle*

(c) a tourniquet may be used to locate the vein and for the introduction of the needle. *Before* the blood sample is taken the tourniquet should be *released*, for venous congestion may lead to errors of up to 10% in for instance haematocrit and plasma protein

(d) *forearm exercise* before taking blood may lead to falsely high $[K^+]$ values

(e) blood should not be squirted though a fine needle into the sample bottle—this may cause *haemolysis*

(f) for *blood gas estimations* to be of any value, the blood must at all times be protected from air. Blood (usually arterial) should be collected in a heparinized disposable syringe, the needle stopped with a cork or the syringe capped and immediately transported to the laboratory

(g) *speed* in the sample reaching the laboratory is of importance.

2. *Laboratory errors.* In general these are of three types:

(a) *random:* these may be human or technical and occur with a frequency inversely proportional to the quality of the laboratory. Autoanalysers have greatly reduced the sources of random error, but no laboratory is yet entirely free from them

(b) *systematic:* these too have been greatly reduced by means of autoanalysers, especially by their sophisticated inbuilt quality control systems, and by accompanying computer data-storage and retrieval systems that allow a much more exact determination of what range of values should be regarded as normal for a particular investigation, in a patient of a particular age and sex, in a particular hospital

(c) *statistical:* there is a further source of error, the origin of which lies partly in the laboratory and partly in the mind of the clinician who interprets the laboratory result. The normal reference ranges of values are usually constructed by the laboratory for each individual test and usually represent 95% confidence or tolerance limits but they are uncorrected for age or sex and include all 'abnormal' values. The statistical problem is that one time in 20 it is to be expected that a 'normal' person will have a value for the test that is outside the reference range. The risk of this occurrence is greatly magnified when a biochemical or haematological profile containing 12 to 20 items is carried out.

THE IMPORTANCE OF THESE SOURCES OF ERROR IS THAT A MAJOR DECISION WHICH DEPENDS ON A SINGLE LABORATORY RESULT, PARTICULARLY WHEN IT IS UNEXPECTED, SHOULD NEVER BE TAKEN WITHOUT REPEATING THE ESTIMATION.

3. *Errors of interpretation.* With increasing systematisation of sampling, automation of laboratory tests and the printout of their results, sampling and laboratory errors have been greatly reduced. However, automation has also brought with it a vastly greater capacity to generate laboratory data and has accentuated another source of error—interpretation of data by the clinician. Instead of being presented with laboratory information bit by bit, he is now faced with large chunks, and for the most part finds difficulty in interpreting these in relation to the symptoms and signs that the particular patient exhibits. At the same time the clinician is burdened with the enormous growth in quantity of other sorts of data, derived from radiological, radionuclide, ultrasonic, thermographic, and similar tests, each with its own unique sources of technical and interpretive error. To these must be added the dimension of time, within which the patient, his disease, his doctor, and these numerical and graphical data vary.

There is little doubt that the solution to this new problem of information overload lies in the generator of the problem: the computer. Regrettably, computer-assisted medical decision-making is still in its infancy, and progress has lagged far behind the capacity to generate new data. But between this edition and the next it can be anticipated that house surgeons will be gaining computer-assistance of this kind. (We said this in the last edition and we continue to live in hope.)

LABORATORY NOMENCLATURE AND METRIC (SI) UNITS

The house surgeon should be aware of the changes that are taking place in laboratory nomenclature, especially that used for enzymic estimations. Clinical biochemists, like most mortals, are finding it difficult to arrive at international agreement about the nomenclature and methods of estimating enzymic activity: as an Appendix we have listed some of the enzymic estimations in common use, and what has become the agreed nomenclature and abbreviations.

The house surgeon will also be aware that what he thought was the metric system has changed. In the Système Internationale (SI) there are no longer milliequivalents but millimoles; no longer mmHg but kilopascals; and so forth. Because of the confusion that necessarily accompanies change, we have included a further Appendix containing a tabular account of the SI system and the corresponding abbreviations.

REFERENCE VALUES

'Normality' must refer to a subset of the population which is to be tested for 'abnormality'. Thus normal values determined, for instance, from a population of healthy medical students or nurses are quite meaningless if applied to an inpatient hospital population. Because of the not inconsiderable difficulty of defining a 'normal' inpatient, the term 'reference value' or 'reference range' is now often used.

In any biological system or population there is variance, so that no single numerical value can be referred to as an index of normality. In practice, therefore, laboratories provide a reference range of values, within which 90 or 95% of values obtained from the reference 'normal' population will lie. An abnormal value can be defined simply as one that lies outside this range. With more precision the degree of deviation from the reference range can be indicated on a percentile basis.

The reference range must incorporate not merely the biological variance in the population being tested, but also all sampling and laboratory errors which are obtained in everyday practice. Quite evidently, the methods of measurement used in a laboratory, and the units in which the results are expressed, will also affect the numerical values of reference ranges.

From the above it is clear that the reference ranges of laboratory values are unique to your own hospital laboratory and hospital population. In hospitals that use automated techniques laboratory results are printed out by computer, together with the reference range for the particular hospital population, and an index of the deviation of the individual results from the reference range. There is little purpose, therefore, in continuing to provide a table of 'normal' values within this text. As an Appendix at the end, reference values from the Institute of Medical and Veterinary Science of South Australia are given in order to provide a general idea of normality.

MICROBIOLOGY

General

Microbiology laboratories usually perform the following tests:

(a) microscopy and culture for bacteria, fungi and viruses
(b) sensitivity tests
(c) serology or antibody estimations
(d) antibiotic assays.

Treatment of infections requires a knowledge of the infecting organisms and samples, for microscopy and culture, must be taken before antibiotic therapy is begun. When specimens are collected it is important to avoid contamination: skin must be thoroughly disinfected before taking blood cultures (organic iodine preparations are best) and the vulva or penis must be cleansed before collection of mid-stream urines. Swabs from infected wounds or sinuses may give false results because of superficial colonizing bacteria. This problem can be minimised by removing surface debris with sterile saline or aspirating pus into a syringe.

Once specimens are collected they must be transported within 2 hours to the laboratory. Out-of-hours, or if a longer delay is envisaged, special transport media, such as Stewarts, should be used for swabs, urine should be refrigerated and in some circum- stances (e.g. whooping cough) it will be necessary to plate out material on to special agar for incubation. Many infections involve fastidious organisms such as obligate anaerobic *Bacteroides fragilis* in appendicitis, *Chlamydia trachomatis* in pelvic inflammatory disease and gonococci. Special swabs and transport systems are provided by the laboratory for fastidious organisms. You should acquaint yourself with these systems in your hospital and also learn how to 'plate out' after hours if this facility is available.

Emergency tests can be done in life-saving or unusual circumstances. Microscopic examination of inflammatory exudates, and occasionally blood cultures, will often indicate the species of organism most likely to be involved rapid; serological tests can be used to diagnose serum hepatitis, syphilis and bacterial meningitis. Culture and sensitivity results take at least 24 hours.

The information provided on the request form will often determine how a specimen is processed and results are interpreted. For example, *Staphylococcus epidermidis* in a blood culture might be a contaminant but if the patient is known to have a prosthetic heart valve or a central venous line the organism will be considered as significant and sensitivity tests undertaken. The laboratory cannot be expected to provide full interpretation of all results and the microbiologist should be consulted whenever dubious results are obtained or assistance with diagnosis is required.

HISTOLOGY AND MORBID ANATOMY

Every operation specimen must be sent to the pathologist for histological examination. You must ask when *not* to obtain histology not the converse. When the result is required within 2-3 days the request form should be marked 'urgent'. *Frozen sections* are undertaken by special prearrangement. Some laboratories operate a 'rapid turnround' system by which a specimen delivered (say) by 09.30 is reported on by 16.30. This can be very useful in scheduling operations for breast lumps where preoperative diagnosis of cancer obtained by using a needle biopsy may make a frozen section unnecessary.

A frequent problem is that specimens are not sent to the pathologist in prime condition. There are usually local rules, but the following are always applicable:

1. Mucosal biopsies (e.g. from the colon or rectum) are pressed out onto a piece of thick card before being immersed in fixative. This helps the pathologist to orientate them and stops them curling up. Lymph node biopsies, especially where lymphomas are suspected, are best prepared by immediate imprint of the transversely cut surface on to a glass slide which is air dried. The cut

node is then immersed in 10% formalin.

2. Organ specimens should be pinned out on cork. A salient point such as the apex of a dissection for cancer is identified by a marker—a black, silk stitch does very well—and this fact mentioned in the request form.

3. If a hollow viscus has not been emptied or opened, consider whether you need to insert preservative into the lumen to ensure even fixation.

4. Whenever possible avoid these problems by delivering specimens yourself.

Remember that you are obtaining an opinion from a consultant, and he cannot give help unless *full clinical details* including the existence of previous biopsies are supplied on the request form.

5. If a pathological specimen has been obtained elsewhere tell the pathologist and he will obtain blocks and/or a report.

HAEMATOLOGY

Haematological screening has now also become automated, mainly by way of cell counters and sizers, so that a much more comprehensive set of cell counts, sizes, types, and content is now available on a routine basis, often with a computer-printed diagnosis or suggestion for further investigation. Nevertheless, if the result seems unusual, or is not susceptible to full interpretation, do not hesitate to *consult with the haematologist.*

Chapter 5

Special Investigations

GASTRIC SECRETORY FUNCTION TESTS

There is little indication for these tests in the routine diagnosis of gastric or duodenal ulcer, but they may be of value in three circumstances:

1. In patients suspected of having the Zollinger–Ellison syndrome.
2. In the diagnosis of pernicious anaemia.
3. The investigation of patients with recurrent dyspepsia after surgical treatment.

These tests measure the amount of hydrochloric acid secreted over a period of time or as a result of a stimulus. It is desirable to know the absolute quantity of acid secreted, which is the product of the concentration and volume. All depend on the proper placement of the gastric tube. Whenever possible a Salem double lumen tube size 14 or 16 French gauge should be inserted into the stomach so that free aspiration of gastric juice is obtained. For reliable results the patient should be supervised throughout the test by a trained nurse or a doctor.

Maximum Stimulation Tests

The stomach can be made to secrete acid to its maximum by using either histamine or a synthetic gastrin (the penta–peptide pentagastrin). The latter is now used as it avoids the very slight possibility of reaction to histamine. The test gives a rough measure of parietal cell mass and is thus useful in determining whether the patient is in the 'duodenal ulcer range' and possibly also in assessing patients after surgery.

All antacids and H_2–receptor antagonist drugs should be withheld for at least 24 hours prior to the test. The patient is fasted for 12 hours and the gastric tube is inserted. *Basal secretion* is collected by continuous gastric aspiration for a period of 60 minutes. Thereafter pentagastrin 6 µg/kg IM is given and the gastric aspirate is collected every 15 minutes for a further 60 minutes. *The maximal acid output* is the quantity of acid contained in the two consecutive 15 minute collections which have the highest acid output. This result is multiplied by two. Typical results in mmol/h of hydrochloric acid are shown in Table 1.

Table 1

Normal		Gastric ulcer		Duodenal ulcer		Pernicious anaemia	
BAO	MAO^{PG}	BAO	MAO^{PG}	BAO	MAO^{PG}	BAO	MAO^{PG}
Men							
2–4	25–45	0.5–3	15–35	3–6	30–60	0	0–0.25
Women							
1–3	20–40	0.5–2	10–25	3–5	25–50	0	0–0.25

BAO = Basal acid output (mmol/h)
MAO^{PG} = Maximal pentagastrin stimulated output (mmol/h)

Note: Though pentagastrin is given in a dose of 6 µg/kg body weight in patients before gastric surgery, after a vagotomy has been performed the dose is increased to 10 µg/kg.

1) These are average values and figures outside these ranges have little diagnostic significance in individual patients.
2) In patients who hypersecrete acid, the Zollinger–Ellison syndrome should be suspected if the basal acid output exceeds 50% of the maximal stimulated output.

Insulin Test Meal (modified Hollander)

The test was developed to assess the completeness of vagotomy. It is difficult to perform and even more difficult to interpret. It is no longer recommended.

LIVER FUNCTION TESTS

All jaundiced patients must have their status for hepatitis B determined and, until this is proved negative, special precautions in handling their blood are in order. In some units patients from high-risk areas (e.g. Africa, Middle East) or from high-risk groups (intravenous drug abusers and male homosexuals) are also screened.

Those tests most useful in surgical practice, and to be applied to every jaundiced patient, are:

> serum bilirubin concentration
> serum alkaline phosphatase (ALP)
> serum transaminase (AST)
> serum albumin (and total protein)
> prothrombin time or index

The most sensitive of the above tests to indicate hepatocellular damage is the AST level. While the concentration will steadily rise with increasing duration of bile duct obstruction, levels in excess of 500 i.u./l almost always indicate hepatitis and should be a warning against accepting a diagnosis of extrahepatic obstruction without other clear-cut evidence. The above liver function tests, although sometimes providing a clear-cut differentiation between a medical and surgical cause for jaundice, may be misleading as there is substantial overlap between results for individual tests in various medical and surgical conditions. Another useful screening test is abdominal ultrasound imaging which can, in many instances, provide confirmation of a diagnosis made on the basis of clinical examination and blood tests. (See the management of jaundice p.171.)

Liver function tests have a wider role than merely investigating the patient who is presumed to have liver disease. They can *screen* for alcoholism when the glutamyl transferase is often raised; they are essential in the management of parenteral nutrition (p.97); and the albumin level may be of use in nutritional deficiency, renal disease and in allowing standardisation of serum calcium concentration. Gamma glutaryl transferase is a sensitive index of liver damage by alcohol.

CANCER ANTIGENS

Thus far, three classes of proteins released into the blood stream by cancers, and detectable by immunological means, have been recognised to have some diagnostic value. One is the *alpha-fetoprotein* (or *globulin*), which appears in the plasma in quantities of mg/ml in about 85% of persons who develop hepatocellular carcinoma. The test has a low false-positive rate. Alpha-fetoprotein may also be produced by malignant teratomas of the testis or ovary, when the plasma level may be of value in monitoring the response to therapy.

The second is the *carcinoembryonic antigen (CEA)*, present in ng/ml amounts in patients with a variety of cancers: in particular, those of the large bowel, pancreas, lung, breast and urinary tract. It is also present in some patients with alcoholic cirrhosis, pancreatitis, and some apparently normal persons. Few laboratories have established proper tolerance limits for plasma CEA in non-cancerous patients. However, at best the clinical value for plasma CEA estimation as a diagnostic test for cancer is low, because a 70–80% false negative rate is necessary in order to achieve a false positive rate as low as 5%. In cancer patients with elevated levels at the time of initial diagnosis and treatment, serial CEA estimations are used as a guide to persistence or recurrence of tumour.

The third group are the *human chorionic gonadotropins* secreted by testicular teratoma and chorion epithelioma. They are relatively specific and baseline values should be obtained to control therapy.

Monoclonal antibodies against tumour antigens are under continuous development and show some promise for the future.

OTHER ANTIGENS AND AUTOANTIBODIES

Blood tests for a variety of other antigens and antibodies are now fairly freely available. In many cases their diagnostic value is not yet numerically defined, but a list is appended, together with conditions in which they may be positive:

Thyroid antibodies
   thyroid microsomal   }   Hashimoto's disease
   thyroglobulin   }   Primary myxoedema
   thyroid stimulating
     immunoglobulin (TSIg)   Graves' disease

Gastric antibodies
  parietal cell
  intrinsic factor }
	Pernicious anaemia

Adrenal antibodies	Idiopathic (non-tuberculous) Addison's disease

Antibodies in liver disease
  smooth muscle
	Chronic active hepatitis
	  (if HBsAg negative)

mitochondrial	Primary biliary cirrhosis

Hepatitis antigens/antibodies
  hepatitis B surface antigen
  (HBsAg)
	Hepatitis B or carrier state

hepatitis B antibody
  (anti HBs)
	Indicative of past infection
	  with HB virus

IgM hepatitis B core antibody
  (IgM anti HB_c)
	Indicates recent
	  infection or continuing
	  viral replication in the liver

hepatitis Be antigen and
  antibody
  (HB_eAg and anti HB_e)
	Only in HBsAg positive sera,
	  the former indicates high
	  infectivity

IgM antibody to hepatitis A
  virus
	Specific for recent infection
	  with HA virus

Reticulin antibodies	Coeliac disease, dermatitis herpetiformis
Glomerular basement membrane antibodies	Goodpasture's syndrome
Skin intercellular antibody	Pemphigus
Skin basement membrane antibody	Pemphigoid
Striated muscle antibodies	Myasthenia gravis
Acetylcholine esterase receptor antibodies	Myasthenia gravis
Rheumatoid factor(s)	Rheumatoid arthritis
Antinuclear antibodies	Various connective tissue diseases including SLE

Native DNA antibodies	Systemic lupus erythematosus (SLE)
Antibodies to extractable nuclear antigens (ENA)	Various connective tissue diseases, high titre anti–RNP antibody particularly characteristic of mixed connective tissue disease
Anti-HIV (HTLV III) antibody	Pre-AIDS (acquired immunodeficiency syndrome) and AIDS.

URINARY TRACT

Urine Specimens

In order to obtain an adequate mid–stream urine specimen the patient must have a full bladder (i.e. preferably early morning) and pass some 200 ml of urine to wash out urethral organisms before the sterile container is placed in the uninterrupted stream.

Male: the prepuce must be retracted and the glans washed with sterile saline.

Female: the patient inserts a vaginal tampon and holds the labia apart with her fingers. She then cleans the periurethral region with sterile saline, collects the specimen and removes the tampon.

Catheter specimens may introduce infection, and contamination with urethral organisms makes bacteriological interpretation difficult. They should be used only when a patient is unable to cooperate.

The risk of catheter-induced infection can be reduced by instilling 50 ml of 0.2% neomycin solution before removing the catheter.

The specimen should reach the laboratory within *one hour*. Out of hours, specimens will keep in the refrigerator (not the ice compartment!) overnight.

1. Microscopical examination for *red cells, pus cells* and *casts.* When chronic pyelonephritis is sought, a *quantitative white cell count* may be valuable—WBC excretion should be <100 000/h; >200 000/h is abnormal.

Phase-contrast microscopy distinguishes *glomerular bleeding* (a pleomorphic pattern, found with the low counts of normal subjects or with high counts in nephritis) from *non-glomerular* or *surgical bleeding* (an isomorphic pattern which is always abnormal and demands urological investigation).

Bladder urine should be sterile. Though the presence of $>10^5$ colony-forming units/ml is a useful index of infection in epidemiological studies, this criterion is too insensitive for the individual patient. In a well-collected specimen (especially in males) a lower count may indicate infection.

2. *Quantitative bacterial culture* and assessment of in vitro *antibiotic sensitivities*. Bacterial count should be $<10\,000$ organisms/ml; $>100\,000$/ml is definitely abnormal, *provided* less than 1 hour has elapsed after voiding.

Bladder Cytology

Cytological examination of the urine has proved of some value in the investigation of suspected bladder carcinoma. Specimens should *not* be early morning ones. An equal volume of 10% formalin is added *at once*. Cytology is also useful in follow-up of patients with bladder cancer. For best results the voided urine should be collected directly into formalin to preserve cell morphology.

Measurement of Renal Function

1. *Serum creatinine* concentration is a simple and reasonably reliable measure of renal function. Blood urea concentration is affected by many other factors, including protein intake and hydration. Serum creatinine only rises, however, when there has been substantial nephron loss.

2. *Creatinine clearance* is a reasonably good guide to glomerular filtration rate. It is best measured on a 24-hour urine specimen. The patient empties the bladder on waking, discards the urine, and enters the time on the collection bottle. All urine is then collected up to and including a specimen 24 hours later. A blood sample for serum creatinine concentration is taken during the collection period.

Prostatic Biopsy

This, by the transrectal or transperineal route, has replaced prostatic massage as the method of obtaining a diagnosis in prostatic cancer. The simplest and easiest method is to aspirate cells by the transrectal route (see p.193).

ENDOSCOPY

All house staff should be able to pass a proctoscope and a sigmoidoscope. They should also know the indications and methods of preparation for more complicated endoscopic examinations (Table 2).

Proctoscopy

A proctoscope is a short, wide, open-ended tube through which the anal canal and lower few centimetres of the rectum can be examined. Built-in illumination is normally provided. No special preparation or anaesthesia is required. The knee–chest position is best, but the lateral position is more usual. A digital examination is made first and the patient then told to expect an instrument of approximately the same size. Do not proceed if the digital examination causes severe pain. The instrument with its obturator in place is warmed, lubricated, and gently introduced to its full length, pointing at the umbilicus. The obturator is then removed. First inspect the rectal mucosa for colour (salmon pink is normal), rugosity, ulceration, excess mucus and redundancy of folds. Then withdraw the instrument slowly, observing for piles and their prolapse through the sphincter.

Sigmoidoscopy

Most diagnostic sigmoidoscopes are about 25–30 cm in length and up to 2 cm in diameter. They are hollow tubes with an obturator and a light source, which may be proximal, distal, or best of all fibreoptic. No special preparation of the patient is necessary nor indeed desirable beyond possibly mild sedation. The left lateral position with the hips well flexed and raised on a pillow is best. The instrument should be warm, well lubricated and introduced to 5 cm pointing at the umbilicus. Then remove the obturator and advance the instrument under vision. In the lateral position a plain lens and air-insufflator are used to open up the lumen ahead of the instrument. If you encounter faeces, sneak the instrument alongside rather than trying to clean them out. Alternatively, give a disposable enema and repeat the examination. Considerable experience, skill, and care may be required to get round the rectosigmoid junction; in about half the patients this is impossible. Interpretation of what you see also requires experience.

Table 2 Endoscopic procedures

Endoscope	Range of instrument	Diagnostic applications	Therapeutic applications	Preparation
Proctoscope	Anal canal Ano-rectal junction	Haemorrhoids, fissure, fistula, proctitis	Injection of haemorrhoids	Nil
Sigmoidoscope	Rectum Lower 1/3 sigmoid	Diffuse mucosal changes (proctitis, colitis) Discrete lesions (polyp, cancer)	Removal of polyps Release of sigmoid volvulus Fulguration or cryo-destruction of cancer (palliative)	Nil or disposable enema
Flexible sigmoidoscope	Mid-descending colon	Investigation of bleeding and obstructive symptoms	Polypectomy (occasionally)	Disposable enema cathartic
Colonoscope	Whole colon	As above	Removal of polyps Decompression in pseudo-obstruction	Cathartic
Oesophagoscope	Oesophagus	Oesophagitis, stricture, cancer, foreign body	Dilation of stricture Removal of foreign body	Nil by mouth for 8 hours

Instrument	Access	Diagnostic	Therapeutic	Preparation / Anaesthesia
Gastro-duodenoscope	Stomach (except close to cardia) All the duodenum including papilla	Diffuse mucosal changes (varices, gastritis, erosions, linitis plastica) Discrete lesions (ulcer, cancer, polyp) Obstructive jaundice Duodenal biopsy for small bowel disease	Laser coagulation of bleeding vessels Removal of common duct stones	Nil by mouth 8 hours ERCP: ? Vitamin K ? Prophylactic antibiotics
Choledochoscope	Common bile and hepatic ducts	Exclusion of calculi	—	Remind operating room
Laparoscope	Liver, gall bladder, spleen Ovaries, tubes, rectovaginal pouch Appendix	Liver tumours, peritoneal metastases Acute abdomen	Tubal destruction	? General anaesthesia If so appropriate arrangements
Cystoscope	Bladder, bladder neck, urethra	Inflammation, tumour, stone, injury Retrograde urography	Fulguration tumour Extraction ureteric stone	Usually general anaesthesia
Resectoscope	Bladder, bladder neck, posterior urethra	As above	Resection prostate, bladder neck, bladder tumour	Usually spinal anaesthesia
Rigid and flexible bronchoscope	Down to orifices of third order bronchi	Mucosal lesions (cancer) Compressive lesions (nodes) Origin of pus or blood	Bronchial toilet	Remind nursing staff of problems with anaesthetised vocal cords

Chapter 6

Imaging

Because one of the surgeon's main concerns is what is inside the patient's body, imaging is central to his diagnostic and therapeutic role. House surgeons will spend a great deal of time requesting and arranging various kinds of imaging (and regrettably also in many hospitals a lot of effort in finding the results when they are needed) so that a firm grasp of the principles of application of imaging to surgical circumstances is essential.

REQUESTING THE INVESTIGATION

The following questions are relevant.

1. Is this a request I can make or do I need clearance from someone more senior?

2. Am I sure that I have selected the most appropriate investigation?

3. Because of 1. and 2., do I need to make a personal approach to the individual who will undertake and/or interpret the images?

4. Have I filled in the form correctly and with sufficient detail about the objectives of the test?

5. Have I found all the previous relevant images and indicated when complementary images are available?

6. Do I need to accompany the patient (e.g. with a head injury or a compromised airway)?

7. Do I need to be there when the technique is being deployed (see for example p. 212)?

CHOICE OF TECHNIQUE

This is a matter of balancing a complex equation of cost, hazard and diagnostic precision. Circumstances always determine cases but the following may be helpful.

Conventional radiology. This is still the mainstay of imaging but is rapidly becoming integrated with other techniques. Its disadvantages are cost and the risks associated with ionising radiation. The latter increases the individual's chance of malignant disease and also affects genetic tissue in ovary and testis. Thus, any x-ray examination, and in particular repeated examinations (e.g. routine daily chest films in patients in the ITU), should not be ordered without some awareness of these small but real risks. The fetus is regarded as being at special risk in the first few weeks of its existence when a woman may not even be aware that she is pregnant. Nearly all departments of radiology have a policy which avoids non-urgent x-rays in women of child-bearing age except in the 14 days following the onset of menstruation.

Two developments of conventional radiology have become of great importance. The first is computerised tomography (CT) which can be used

1. As a plain radiograph to give a cross section of any level of the body (but usually only head, neck and trunk)
2. With two different types of contrast enhancement
    (a) gastrointestinal with water soluble contrast medium taken orally
    (b) intravascular contrast given intravenously and designed to show vascular channels.

CT is expensive but can be crucial in imaging the central nervous system, for example in the evaluation of head injuries. It is also still the most precise way of outlining soft tissue masses and has numerous specialised applications such as sizing abdominal aneurysms and detecting occult metastases in liver and lymph nodes.

Digital subtraction angiography is another development of conventional contrast radiology. An x-ray is taken of the area of interest. Contrast medium is then injected and further exposures made. The 'background' of the plain film is then subtracted electronically leaving the area which contains the contrast (the vascular system) highlighted. The advantages lie not only in the possibility of using less contrast, sometimes injected intravenously rather than intra-arterially but also in more precise imaging. Digital subtraction has replaced conventional arteriography in many circumstances.

Ultrasound. This technique has, so far as is known, no deleterious biological effects. It is also cheaper in some of its applications and thus is gaining ground in a number of areas as the primary method of imaging, particularly if repeated assessment is required. It has three drawbacks the latter two of which are often underestimated by its proponents.

1. It is clearly inapplicable to body sites where there is a bony shield—the head, chest and to a lesser extent the pelvis.

2. Much of the work is done by the ultrasonographer manipulating a surface probe to build up a static image which can then be stored. This means that the technique is operator dependent and operators do vary in their skills and experience.

3. The images produced by ordinary ultrasound are much more difficult for the surgeon to understand than conventional x-rays and many clinicians are hesitant to accept the ultrasongrapher's explanation of what seems little more than a blur.

This having been said, ultrasonography is very useful in delineating masses, outlining soft tissues and contrasting these with calcification or stones, and in assessing progress. Dynamic or 'real time' ultrasound is a more specialised technique with its principal applications at the moment in the cardiovascular system.

Ultrasound can also be very useful in obtaining a 'guided biopsy' of a deep mass in the neck, chest and abdomen.

Radionuclide imaging. The same biological problems apply as with x-rays though the hazards are vanishingly small. Anatomically it is less precise but its great advantage is that in many instances it can be made

1. dynamic
2. specific.

An example of the first is biliary excretion scanning in detecting a non-functional gall bladder or delayed excretion of bile in early obstructive jaundice. An instance of the second is the use of indium-labelled leucocytes to detect and define a septic focus. Bone scintiscanning is also of value in screening patients who are suspected of having metastatic bone involvement.

Scintiscanning was first introduced in the thyroid but now has relatively little application there provided good quality ultrasound is available.

REGIONAL APPLICATIONS

A set of applications which must necessarily be incomplete is given here because we know of no other place in which it is possible to find a concise vade mecum which can help the houseman.

Head

Plain radiography will detect most skull fractures, pneumatoceles and calcified intracranial lesions. There is debate about whether every head-injured patient should have a skull x-ray, but comatose patients with a skull fracture have a 40% chance of a localised intracranial haematoma so a liberal policy should be used. Conventional and Townes (through the orbit from below) views should be requested. If available, CT is mandatory for the comatose head injury and also if any neurological deterioration occurs in a previously well patient.

Head CT is often used in patients

1. with suspected metastases to the brain
2. who are at risk of or who have already had a stroke.

Scintiscanning may also detect brain metastases but otherwise has limited diagnostic utility.

Subtraction angiography is used in intra- and extracranial vascular disease.

NMR scanning of the brain gives superior or unique information in many circumstances.

Cervical Spine

In suspected bone injury, great care should be taken both in carrying out x-rays and in interpreting them. AP, lateral and odontoid views are usually ordered. The houseman is advised never to risk interpretation even in a preliminary way and always to seek advice.

Facial Bones

Do not merely ask for x-ray of facial bones but request views of the bone thought to be fractured, e.g. zygoma, maxilla, mandible or the regions of interest, such as the paranasal sinuses.

Ribs and Sternum

Though the diagnosis of fracture of both these is clinical, a chest x-ray gives some indication of the extent of rib damage and thus of the need for ventilatory support. The additional advantage of a chest film is that it can show internal damage—contusion, pneumothorax, fluid in the chest and mediastinal widening.

Trunk Bones

A common indication here, as in other bony sites, is to check a 'hot spot' revealed by scintiscanning in a patient suspected of having bone disease (usually metastatic cancer). The radiographer never and the radiologist seldom has the scan available, so it is doubly important that you tell them on the request form where exactly the suspicious area is thought to be.

In trauma, PA and lateral views are required for the thoraco-lumbar spine, but an AP is initially adequate for the pelvis. Laterals can be obtained later for the doubtful case.

Neck

For thyroid and other neck swellings, ultrasound is the first investigation. It will nearly always distinguish cystic from solid lesions and may give additional information about the rest of the gland or detect other lumps outside it. Preoperatively, a plain x-ray will demonstrate deviation or compression of the trachea, information that is particularly useful to the anaesthetist. Uptake scans are needed only in special circumstances though they tend still to be ordered.

Breast

Though many other ways than the use of x-rays have been sought to image the breast, mammography remains the most used. Technique has improved so that the radiation dose is acceptable. Mammography's uses are:

1. Screening in high risk patients.

2. Study of the contralateral breast in patients with cancer.

3. Rarely for the investigation of a 'doubtful' breast lump. In that all breast lumps should be examined cytologically or histopathologically, mammography for this purpose should seldom be used.

Chest

Probably one of the commonest exposures made on surgical patients. Lateral films rarely should be requested. Erect films are the only satisfactory ones. Supine views are useless, except in patients on mechanical ventilation, when the exposure can be made at the peak of inspiration. You must personally make sure that the patient is at least sat up. Even very ill patients can be held momentarily erect.

Abdomen

There is controversy now about whether erect as distinct from supine views of the abdomen have any role in diagnosis, especially in intestinal obstruction. Some departments are loath to provide them. However, they are occasionally useful in a doubtful case of small bowel obstruction and should be requested when this condition is a possibility. Plain x-rays are quite unnecessary when the clinical diagnosis is acute appendicitis, salpingitis or other infective-inflammatory conditions. They are also quite unreliable in showing gas under the diaphragm for which an erect chest x-ray should be taken. Lateral films of the abdomen are not often indicated but may sometimes reveal the calcified edge of an aortic aneurysm.

The presence of an abdominal mass may be an indication for an ultrasound or a CT scan or may call for some form of contrast radiography. Consult before ordering these investigations.

Even when a mass is not present, both scanning techniques have their use in detecting liver metastases (on balance CT is superior to ultrasound), organ enlargement (e.g. liver, spleen, pancreas, kidney) and occult collections of fluid or abscesses.

Gastrointestinal Tract

Classical contrast examination is by the use of barium. However, the widespread use of flexible endoscopy at both ends (see p.52) enables direct vision of the upper tract as far as the third part of the duodenum and of the lower tract to the ileocaecal valve. Biopsies can also be taken to give a pathological diagnosis or to chart the extent of, say, an inflammatory process. In consequence, the balance between radiology and endoscopy is altering and routine use of the former becoming less. Reflect therefore, before ordering contrast studies, whether they are going to give as much information as might endoscopy. For precise delineation of the small bowel a 'barium meal and follow through' is inappropriate. A small bowel 'enema' after duodeno-jejunal intubation is the correct investigation. For examination of the large bowel, double contrast (air and barium) is the only acceptable standard though even this is inferior to colonoscopy in the detection of polyps.

Water soluble contrast examination (the usual agent is Gastrografin) has a variety of uses:

1. To establish that the gastrointestinal tract is functioning, e.g. after surgery.

2. To detect a leak from either a perforation or a suture line. The reliability of this is not perfect and the absence of radiological demonstration does not imply that all is necessarily well.

3. To confirm or confute the presence of intestinal obstruction:
   (a) when small bowel obstruction is a possibility 50-100 ml of contrast medium can be given orally and films exposed at 5 minutes, 1 hour, and if there is still doubt, after 4 hours. This is by no means a routine practice and should only be done under supervision.
   (b) if large bowel obstruction is a possibility but the patient may also be at risk from pseudo-obstruction (and this confusion is quite likely in elderly patients who may be hypoxic, uraemic, anaemic or bed-ridden—all of which predispose to the condition), then a water soluble contrast enema is very useful in preventing an unnecessary operation and, less commonly but also importantly, sometimes demonstrating that the diagnosis is not pseudo-obstruction but an organic cause.

Biliary Tree

In acute abdominal pain of possible biliary origin, ultrasound is the currently popular initial investigation and has replaced to a very great extent the use of oral cholecystography which is unreliable. Ultrasound will show:

1. Biliary calculi in the gall bladder and biliary tree.
2. A distended and/or thick-walled gall bladder.
3. Dilated ducts if these are present.
4. In skilled hands abnormalities in the pancreatic head.

In jaundiced patients ultrasound can:
1. Demonstrate dilated ducts, which is the cardinal sign that the jaundice is post-hepatic.
2. Demonstrate calculi.
3. In skilled hands show ductal or pancreaticoduodenal lesions causing the jaundice.

On the outcome of ultrasound is predicated the choice of further investigations to give a precise anatomical diagnosis. In the jaundiced patient invasive investigations are not undertaken without considering:
1. The bleeding risk—is the prothrombin time normal? Even if it is, it is good practice to prescribe vitamin K in any patient who has been jaundiced for more than 2 weeks.
2. Is antibiotic prophylaxis indicated?

In non-jaundiced patients, and if the diagnosis on ultrasound is unequivocally gall stones, many surgeons will not ask for further investigation. Intravenous cholegraphy is thus less commonly used which may be a good thing because it does carry slight risks of hypersensitivity to the relatively large dose of contrast medium which is used. However, it has the advantage that it bypasses the absorption process in the gastrointestinal tract. It can often delineate the anatomy of the biliary tree but with the advent of isotope excretion scanning its role of establishing that there is a non-functioning gall bladder has declined.

In suspected acute cholecystitis or 'biliary colic' when facilities are available an isotope excretion scan (HIDA) can establish that the gall bladder is obstructed or non-functioning with considerable reliability. Many see it as the investigation of choice when the ultrasound is equivocal.

In jaundiced patients the invasive investigations are:

1. From above—percutaneous transhepatic cholegraphy which is safe with a fine needle but may be unsuccessful in outlining a lesion at the lower end of the duct.

2. From below—endoscopic retrograde cholepancreatography (ERCP) which may fail because the ducts cannot be cannulated.

3. Guided biopsy using ultrasound or CT.

4. Angiography—usually arteriography to outline the vascular anatomy of an identified tumour.

Operative cholegraphy is virtually routine throughout the world for operations on the biliary tree.

Renal Tract

A straight film may occasionally help to outline renal abnormalities. More usually, intravenous urography (IVU) remains the best starting point for imaging the renal tract. However, as already indicated, ultrasound may be appropriate for investigating a renal mass. A CT scan and selective angiography are often indicated once a renal mass has been diagnosed. Isotope scanning is occasionally used in special circumstances.

Antegrade pyelography. Under local anaesthesia and using x-ray or ultrasonographic control, a needle can be introduced into the renal collecting system. A guide wire is then fed into the renal pelvis and a track established by passing dilators over the wire. The advantages of this technique are that it does not require a general anaesthetic, the ureter above the point of obstruction can be delineated and, if necessary, a catheter can be left in place to drain a completely or partially obstructed kidney.

Retrograde urography. This way of outlining the upper urinary tract has the disadvantage over antegrade pyelography that a ureteric catheter must be passed via a cystoscope, usually under general anaesthesia and in circumstances where good quality x-rays can be more difficult to obtain. The examination is now only rarely used, because the lower ureter can now be examined directly through an endoscope.

Retrograde urethrography and voiding cystography. Direct cystourethrography is of special value when injury to the urethra or bladder is suspected as in fractured pelvis. However, never pass a catheter in suspected rupture of the urethra without the consent of a senior. The house surgeon may need to make the urethral injection of contrast. If possible the study should be carried out under image intensification so as to minimise extravasation. Cine cystography and urodynamic studies should be arranged only after consultation between radiologists and urologists.

Arterial and Venous Systems

Arteriography. Its applications are to:

1. Show obstruction of the vasculature.

2. Indicate abnormal circulations such as may occur in tumours and congenital malformations.

3. Delineate the vascular anatomy as a guide to planning therapy, e.g. liver resection.

4. Identify an obscure source of bleeding in the gastrointestinal tract.

5. Embolise lesions such as tumours.

6. Follow the dilation of atheromatous strictures by intraluminal balloons.

Arteriography is invasive, though in most instances quite safe. Discussion with the radiologist should usually occur before the investigation is booked. Clinical details should include the site and the nature of the suspected lesion and route suggested (but not demanded) for the injection of the contrast material.

Phlebography. There are two main techniques in the lower limbs.

1. Ascending venography which is used to:

   (a) diagnose deep vein thrombosis and outline its sequelae such as obstruction

   (b) outline the sites of deep to superficial incompetence in complicated varicose vein problems which may be post-phlebitic.

2. Descending venography which is less commonly employed in the post-phlebitic limb.

The indications for venography are complicated and the investigation should not be requested without consultation.

Lymphangiography. This is another highly specialised

investigation. It was formerly used for:

1. Staging abdominal lymphoma.
2. Investigating the lymphoedematous limb.

However, for both circumstances it is now rarely used because it is tedious for the patient and the operator, as well as being relatively insensitive. Isotope lymphography is available in some centres which specialise in lymphatic disorders.

Chapter 7

Blood Transfusion

Stringent regulations for the user of blood and blood products are necessary in order to run an efficient, safe blood transfusion service. For the house surgeon, special attention to blood transfusion procedures is necessary since patients needing urgent surgery are often anaesthetised, or unconscious. Under these conditions the signs of major transfusion reaction may be obscured. The following notes incorporate some guiding principles for house surgeons.

As 'end users' surgeons do not have much to worry about in relation to patients who carry viruses such as those which cause hepatitis B and AIDS. Like others who use a lot of blood, they have a duty not to transfuse irresponsibly as the risks, though very small because of the exemplary standards of blood transfusion services, can never be completely eliminated.

PATIENT IDENTITY

It is essential that a request form for blood or blood products should contain the patient's full name, age or preferably date of birth, hospital identification number, the blood group (if known) and whether or not the person concerned has previously been transfused, has been pregnant, or has known red cell antibodies. Before each unit of blood is given to the patient, the name, hospital number and blood group must be checked with the label on the blood unit; this label should also contain laboratory certification that the blood is compatible with the recipient. These precautions are valueless unless it is certain that the initial blood sample on which cross-matching has been performed was taken from the correct patient. For this reason the house surgeon should either take the blood sample himself, or personally assure himself that the arrangements for blood collection have been carefully carried out according to a written protocol. It is important that specimen containers should not be prelabelled, but should be labelled at the patient's bedside.

It is important to recognise that most major transfusion errors occur as the result of mistakes made in clerical and identification procedures, not from laboratory or technical shortcomings.

REQUESTS FOR BLOOD

Operative procedures can be divided into three categories in which:

1. Blood transfusion is invariable.
2. Blood transfusion is occasional.
3. Blood transfusion is rare.

The house surgeon's aim should be to avoid excessive demands on the transfusion service while ensuring that blood is readily available when required.

These two aims can be reconciled in cases of categories (1) and (2) above by:

1. Sending blood for grouping and antibody screening before the patient is admitted. A good surgical unit will organise this in the outpatient clinic.

2. 48 hours before operation sending a further sample with the appropriate request:

    (a) 'Please cross–match x units of blood for operation on y date'

    or

    (b) 'Please group, antibody screen and hold serum for 3 days'

Cross-matching can be performed on this serum if urgently required.

The safest patient to transfuse is the patient with a negative antibody screen who has never been transfused or had a pregnancy. Transfusion reactions in such patients, except for major ABO incompatibility, are rare.

BLOOD REQUIREMENTS FOR OPERATION

Many hospital blood banks now adopt a policy of grouping, antibody screening and holding serum for cross-matching if required; only for certain specified operative procedures does blood need to be held cross-matched. *In general, blood should not be requested unless it is likely that it will be used.* It is important that the blood bank be informed when blood which has been cross-matched is no longer required, since this allows the blood to be used for another patient or patients. Blood banks will routinely place unused blood back into their unassigned inventory 48 hours after surgery unless specifically requested to keep it in an assigned inventory.

Most hospitals have developed a policy for screening and cross-matching blood for planned surgical procedures. One such list (that at St Mary's Hospital, London) is given below as a guide:

Group and screen only

Amputation
Arthroscopy
Arthrotomy
Bladder tumour: TUR
Cardiac catheter
Cervical rib: inlet explor.
Cervix: cone biopsy
Cholecystectomy; duct explor.
Colostomy; gastrostomy
Cystostomy; cystoscopy
Dilatation and curettage
Embolectomy
Femoral nail: removal
Glossectomy
Hysterectomy
Laminectomy
Laparoscopy
Laparotomy; exploratory
Tubal surgery
Vagotomy and drainage

Mastectomy
Mastoidectomy
Mediastinoscopy
Meniscectomy
Osteotomy: bone biopsy
Ovary: wedge resection
Pacemaker insertion
Palate resection
Parathyroidectomy
Pinning of long bone
Prostatectomy: TUR
Salivary gland removal
Sinus operations
Splenectomy
Sympathectomy: lumbar
Thyroid surgery
Tonsillectomy
Tracheostomy
Ureteric surgery

Group, screen and cross-match 1 unit

Ovarian cystectomy   Pinning fractured neck of femur
(1 unit transfusions are virtually
never justified)

Group, screen and cross-match 2 units

Abdominoperineal resection   Nephrectomy. Graft ditto
Arthroplasty knee/shoulder   Ovarian carcinoma
Atrioventricular septal defect   Patent ductus
Brachial plexus repair   Prostatectomy; open
Fallot's tetralogy   Pyelolithotomy (1st op.)
Hysterectomy (vaginal or abdo.)   Renal transplant
Laryngectomy   Spinal fusion
Mastectomy; radical or lat dorsi   Thoracotomy: pneumonectomy
flap
Maxillectomy   Colectomy
Myomectomy

Group, screen and cross-match 3 units

Adrenalectomy   Hip arthroplasty
Femoropopliteal bypass   Hysterectomy; radical
Gastrectomy; partial   Pulmonary valvotomy

Group, screen and cross-match 4 units

Aortoiliac or femoral bypass   Hip prosthesis
Commando operation   Mitral valve split
Coronary vein graft   Pancreatectomy; partial
Gastrectomy; total   Pyelolithotomy (repeat)

Group, screen and cross-match 6 units

Coronary vein graft (repeat)   Radical cystectomy
Oesophagectomy   Valve replace (1 only)
Pancreatectomy; total   Ventricular aneurysm

Group, screen and cross-match 8 units

Aortic aneurysm; abdominal or   Valve replace (2 or more)
                  thoracic   Vein graft and valve replace

The needs for other operations will be determined by hospital policy.

In replacement of red cells before operation, the transfusion should ideally be given 24–36 hours before surgery to enable the stored cells to recover their full oxygen carrying capacity in vivo. In these patients, reconstituted red cells or packed cells should be used; whole blood is seldom required here.

STORAGE OF BLOOD

All blood must be stored in properly regulated blood bank refrigerators which have visual and audible alarms and a recording chart. The correct temperature for the storage of whole blood, reconstituted red cells and packed cells is 4–6°C. These blood products must never be frozen. Ward refrigerators are unsafe for the storage of blood, particularly if they have a freezing compartment into which blood may inadvertently be placed.

Once units of blood have left the blood bank, unless they are used almost immediately, they may become unsafe if the core temperature of the blood rises above 8°C. In an ambient temperature of 22°C this takes place in 30 minutes. Blood issued from the blood bank should be held in refrigerated insulated containers, and only 1 or 2 units should be issued at a time. If blood is not used, it must be returned immediately to the blood bank. If there is a delay in the return of blood to the blood bank for whatever reason, the packs should be labelled 'Not for transfusion'.

URGENT BLOOD TRANSFUSION

At nights and at weekends in those hospitals where there is not a round the clock blood bank operating, the switchboard operator will have the name and telephone number of the blood bank staff member on duty. Much help can be given in the resolution of clinical problems if early consultation takes place and possible future requests and requirements are explained and discussed personally. This applies particularly in the case of massive transfusion.

The recommended procedure in a patient apparently needing urgent transfusion should be:

1. Warn the blood bank.

2. Insert an IV cannula, using this to take blood samples for grouping, antibody screening and cross-matching.

3. Send or preferably take the sample to the blood bank immediately with the request form.

4. Depending on the degree of urgency, ask for

(a) O Rh(D) negative blood — extreme emergency only (many would say an extreme emergency which necessitates blood as distinct from blood volume expansion justifies ignoring Rhesus status)

(b) Grouped but not cross-matched blood—great urgency—5–10 minutes

(c) Grouped and saline cross-matched blood—15 minutes

(d) Fully cross-matched blood —1–1.5 hours.

5. In the meantime, use a plasma volume expander such as plasma protein solution or a plasma substitute.

At all stages it is essential to weigh the risk of transfusion reaction against that of incomplete or inappropriate replacement of blood loss. It is important to substitute fully cross-matched blood as soon as it becomes available.

Many hospitals now have abbreviated cross-match procedures which allow the earlier safe issue within 20 minutes of blood which has undergone an indirect antiglobulin test. The use of non-cross-matched blood must be kept to an absolute minimum so it is safer to have a simple cross-match done than to have no cross-match at all.

TRANSFUSION REACTIONS

The commonest cause of transfusion reaction in large hospitals these days is a febrile reaction to granulocytes in the multi-transfused individual who has developed white cell antibodies. This type of reaction is very unpleasant and makes the patient feel unwell with headaches and rigors; however, it is rarely dangerous. It must be distinguished from a reaction caused by red cell antibodies, and can be controlled to a certain extent by steroids, but white cell poor blood can be provided by arrangement with the transfusion laboratory. Unfortunately, white cell depletion is a lengthy procedure and can only be performed satisfactorily on blood which is less than 3 days old and so can rarely be provided in an emergency.

Clinically, reactions to red cells may be divided into mild, moderate or severe. All transfusion reactions should be reported to the blood transfusion service.

Mild Reactions

Mild reactions are characterised by transient fever, skin rashes, urticaria and facial oedema. Treatment with antihistamines is usually sufficient. It is usual to discontinue administration of the unit of blood involved and to begin carefully a new unit.

Moderate and Severe Reactions

Any untoward event that occurs during transfusion (fever, rigor, backache, shock) and which suggests incompatibility or bacterial contamination of the blood or blood products must be investigated to determine the cause.

The procedure is as follows:

1. Stop the infusion, keeping all blood units.

2. Re-check all labelling and documentation procedures.

3. Take a specimen of blood into both plain and EDTA tubes, using the arm opposite to that in which transfusion is being given. Send the specimen plus the blood units to the blood bank for appropriate investigations.

4. Always consult with the blood bank staff and the haematologist or pathologist on call. A re-check of the documentation and a repeat cross–match will usually detect if a major serological incompatibility is present and the results of this finding will determine whether urgent further action is required.

5. Observe urinary output carefully.

6. Check the urine for the presence of free haemoglobin.

7. If ABO incompatibility is suspected or confirmed, advise the renal unit promptly.

8. Other laboratory tests which may be of value include the determination of free haemoglobin in serum, plasma haptoglobin and bilirubin levels.

In a well-managed blood bank, major blood group serological reactions are most uncommon. Most transfusion reactions appear to be the result of leucocyte, platelet or plasma antibodies which are often difficult to categorise. If all investigations are negative, cross-matched compatible blood can again be transfused with care, under cover of antihistamines or steroids if required. Febrile reactions which appear to have no specific cause can be treated with antipyretics, but not aspirin.

Severe Reactions

Severe reactions caused by ABO or Rh incompatibility can occur and these are most commonly the consequence of errors in documentation. In any patient in whom severe backache, shock and haemoglobinuria are present, the use of heparin to prevent disseminated intravascular coagulation and infusion of mannitol or intravenous frusemide to promote diuresis should be considered. Such treatment may need to be instituted urgently, but must always be in consultation with the attending clinician, the haematologist and/or pathologist and the renal unit.

BLOOD PRODUCTS AND PLASMA SUBSTITUTES

The availability and cost of blood products varies greatly from country to country and from hospital to hospital. The pattern of usage will depend upon the overall policy applying within the country, the availability of fractionated blood products and the finance available to obtain them.

Whole Blood

Whole blood should be reserved for patients in whom there is acute blood loss and where both red cells and plasma volume replacement are essential. Whole blood should not be used for routine blood transfusion in normovolaemic patients.

Reconstituted Red Cells or Packed Cells (Plasma Depleted Blood)

The recent introduction of red cells resuspended in an electrolyte medium reduces the haematocrit of packed cells and this product is now used in preference to both whole blood and packed cells in many hospitals. The haematocrit is lower than that of packed cells and this results in a better flow rate, comparable with that of whole blood. Reconstituted red cells or packed cells should be used for the management of most patients who require restoration of red cell mass and who are not actively bleeding. Many hospitals now find that over 70% of elective transfusion can be given as packed cells or as reconstituted red cells. This procedure maximises the amount of plasma to be processed into its multiple components. If large amounts of plasma depleted blood are transfused for volume replacement urgently without added electrolyte, then there is a risk that the haemoglobin level will rise above 2.17 mmol/l. This can embarrass the circulation leading to a low output state and oliguria. Check the haemoglobin level urgently after transfusion of more than 4 units of plasma depleted blood.

Platelets

Most centres now prepare platelet concentrates which can be stored for 5 days at room temperature. Platelet-rich plasma, once in common use, is now rarely available. Platelets must be agitated gently during storage and kept at the standard refrigerator temperature. They may be used for the treatment of certain patients with thrombocytopenia and other blood disorders. They may be indicated in the perioperative period as cover for procedures such as splenectomy for thrombocytopenic purpura, portosystemic shunts in patients with liver disease or after massive transfusion. Fresh whole blood (less than 24 hours old) can sometimes be indicated when both platelet and red cell deficiencies are present. It is somewhat of a paradox that in the UK fresh blood is less easily obtainable than platelets.

Leucocyte-poor Red Cells

Various methods are available for the preparation of these, including several different kinds of filter which have largely replaced dextran sedimentation and washing. For patients with repeated transfusion reactions, leucocyte-poor red cells are useful and need to be requested specially from the blood transfusion service.

Plasma Volume Expanders

These can be divided into plasma substitutes and human plasma derivatives. Plasma substitutes include dextran (MW 70 000), modified gelatin ('Haemaccel') and hydroxyethyl starch ('Volex'). All are commercially available and are advantageous as emergency blood volume expanders because of their ready availability, storage characteristics, relatively low cost and freedom from hepatitis and HIV viruses. Each product has advantages and disadvantages, but none is as satisfactory as human plasma derivatives.

Plasma Derivatives

Stable plasma protein solutions (SPPS) obtained by fractionation of human plasma, are now used in many countries. They contain 4–5% protein consisting mainly of albumin with some globulins. The solutions are free of the transmissible viruses and have a long shelf-life. As they are excellent plasma volume expanders they are used extensively in an emergency, but are expensive even in countries where a total voluntary blood donor programme is in place, because of the costs of obtaining and freighting plasma and its subsequent fractionation.

Plasma

Plasma has, in the past, been used as a volume expander but should not be utilised when other safer products are available.

CLOTTING FACTORS AND COAGULATION DEFECTS

In surgical practice it is important to define appropriately any coagulation defects so that proper treatment may be planned. Patients who have a clinical or family history of a bleeding tendency should always be investigated preoperatively in sufficient time to define the defect. Prophylaxis against possible bleeding perioperatively and postoperatively should be planned in consultation with the haematologist.

When a coagulation defect or bleeding diathesis becomes apparent during the course of an operation, the advice of the haematologist may not be available immediately and empirical therapy with clotting factors may be needed. It is advisable in these circumstances to use fresh frozen plasma while remembering that these blood products carry a small but definite risk of transmission of viral diseases. The dangerous situation is a massive transfusion where there may be dilution of clotting factors with subsequent bleeding and oozing.

Two defined clinical circumstances can be described which illustrate the requirements for blood component replacement:

1. In massive blood loss (ruptured aneurysm, major vascular injury, multiple injuries) or blood destruction (prolonged cardio-pulmonary bypass) when many labile clotting factors may be depleted, and there has been massive transfusion, the use of fresh frozen plasma to restore clotting factor levels is advocated. At least 2 units should be given initially. If whole blood is also being used, it may be desirable for it to be less than 10 days from time of collection as this reduces problems associated with microaggregate formation. If there is any evidence of pulmonary insufficiency, a microaggregate filter may be used though its value is questionable. After the transfusion of 10 or more units of blood there is often platelet depletion, and a platelet count and clotting screen should be performed. If the platelet level has fallen below $100 \times 10^9/l$, platelet concentrates may be required.

2. In septicaemia, massive venous thrombosis, brain, prostatic and lung surgery and occasionally in other conditions, coagulation may be followed by excess fibrinolysis with the release of degradation products of fibrin which act as inhibitors of the intrinsic clotting mechanism. Fresh frozen or freeze-dried plasma, often with platelet transfusion, are usually effective so long as the primary condition is adequately controlled. If clotting factor levels are low, the use of cryoprecipitate to provide Factor VIII and fibrinogen may be helpful. On rare occasions an antifibrinolytic agent such as ε-aminocaproic acid (EACA) can be useful.

Consultation with a haematologist is essential for the adequate management of patients with problems such as these.

Chapter 8

IV Fluid Therapy

TECHNIQUES OF IV INFUSION

It is rare nowadays that it is necessary to cut down on a vein. However, patients in shock with a tightly constricted circulation or those with a need for massive transfusion should have a large cannula inserted by exposing a vein in the antecubital fossa. This is preferable to multiple unsuccessful attempts to puncture a vein while the situation is deteriorating. Full aseptic precautions must be observed whenever a cut down is undertaken.

1. Ideally an infusion should not be run into a peripheral vein for more than 24 hours—thrombophlebitis is always painful and sometimes dangerous. Change all peripheral infusions before thrombophlebitis occurs. Although this is a counsel of perfection it *is* possible and, in the long run, saves discomfort for the patient and time for the houseman. Where fluid requirements are not very large 'butterfly' scalp vein needles can be used.
2. Technical points for peripheral infusions:
    (a) become familiar with one piece of equipment and use it all the time
    (b) use the thinnest needle or cannula which will cope with the fluids to be infused
    (c) avoid the elbow fold—that is the antecubital veins. The forearm is best and the dorsum of the hand should only be used as a last resort
    (d) do not use the lower limb—the inevitable immobility and superficial venous thrombosis increase the risk of deep vein thrombosis and pulmonary embolism
    (e) anaesthetise the skin before inserting a catheter by raising an intradermal wheal of 1% lignocaine
    (f) sit down to carry out the venepuncture
    (g) use a tourniquet but do not slap the veins. A gentle tap is enough

(h) do not try to puncture the skin and the vein in one movement. The skin is tough; the vein is not. Puncture the skin to one side of the vein; then take the needle over the vein and deliberately 'dip' into it

(i) secure the cannula yourself. Then you are to blame if it comes out.

3. Central vein infusions are now relatively commonplace, mainly to carry out intravenous feeding. A large variety of cannulae is available and these can be inserted in such a way as to lie in a central vein (usually the brachiocephalic or superior vena cava) so that the administered substances are rapidly diluted by the flow of blood. A long catheter can be led up to the deep veins by percutaneous puncture of the basilic or external jugular vein. The disadvantage of the first is that the arm is immobilised; of the second, that after percutaneous puncture, negotiating the junction of the great veins can be difficult. For these reasons the site of choice is now usually the subclavian below the clavicle, or the internal jugular in the root of the neck. Whether done by percutaneous puncture or direct exposure, this is a job for an expert as the complications are almost endless. Rules to be observed are:

(a) Always take an x-ray after insertion and before starting any infusion to ensure correct placement

(i)   within the vein

(ii) in relation to the chambers of the heart

(iii) to detect the occasional instance when the catheter wanders over to the other side or into the internal jugular vein

(b) Remove the catheter if there is a spike of fever unexplained by any cause. Culture the tip and take a blood culture from a peripheral vein when you do. Catheter-related sepsis may be diagnosed when both the catheter tip and peripheral blood are infected. Some teams use 'draw back' cultures as well and you must be guided by local circumstances

(c) In some units there is a policy of changing the catheter routinely every 7–10 days. However, catheters which are well looked after can stay in for months. If the catheter is to be removed this means complete removal and re-insertion on the opposite side if this is possible

(d) Constantly exhort the nursing staff to the highest standards of sterile procedure in changing the administration apparatus. The best practice now is a 3–litre plastic bag that comes from the pharmacy with a giving set attached. Infusion sets should be changed daily if this service is not available

(e) Change the dressing at the site of catheter entry every second day, cleaning the area with an alcoholic antiseptic such as chlorhexidine. Do not use antibiotic creams because these encourage superinfection

(f) It is standard practice that the catheter used for parenteral nutrition should be regarded as sacrosanct and reserved entirely for this purpose. This means that if a patient is to undergo a major operation or a rapid blood transfusion, an additional catheter of up to 4 mm external diameter should be inserted into an arm vein, following the rules given above. If by necessity a central nutrition catheter is used for other purposes then it should be removed and resited.

Some teams will bend this rule by using a double lumen catheter though experience with this is still limited. Fluids and drugs are infused into the proximal lumen.

INTRAVENOUS SOLUTIONS

We favour the use of simple solutions to which other ingredients can be added at will to suit the needs of individual patients. If such additions make the solution hypertonic then central administration will be required. The electrolyte content and approximate energy value of various solutions are given below:

'Normal' saline	Na^+	150 mmol/l
	Cl^-	150 mmol/l
Hypotonic ('$\frac{1}{5}$th normal') saline and 4% dextrose	Na^+	30 mmol/l
	Cl^-	30 mmol/l
	Calories	140/l (590 kJ/l)
Dextrose 5%	Calories	180/l (756 kJ/l)
'Normal' sodium lactate	Na^+	150 mmol/l
	Lactate$^-$	150 mmol/l
'Normal' sodium bicarbonate	Na^+	150 mmol/l
	HCO_3^-	150 mmol/l
Dextrose 20%	Calories	700/l (2.9 MJ/l)

50% dextrose	Calories	1800/l (70.6 MJ/l)
20% KCl	10 ml =	2 g KCl
		25 mmol/l
Hartmann's balanced salt	Na^+	131 mmol/l
solution	K^+	5 mmol/l
	Ca^{++}	4 mmol/l
	Cl^-	111 mmol/l
	Lactate$^-$	29 mmol/l
Concentrated sodium chloride		Usually supplied
		as 2, 3, or 4
		times 'normal'

5%, 20% and 50% dextrose may also be dispensed with added potassium at varying concentrations.

ALIMENTARY SECRETIONS

As a working rule, the secretions of the alimentary tract can be considered to contain Na^+ 130 mmol/l, K^+ 10 mmol/l, i.e. so far as these cations are concerned each litre lost from the body as vomit, gastrointestinal aspirate, diarrhoea, or from an alimentary fistula may be replaced by a litre of 'normal' saline containing at least 12.5 mmol of K^+.

The situation with regard to anions is more variable: bile, pancreatic juice and small-gut secretions contain large quantities of HCO_3^-, while gastric juice contains large quantities of Cl^-. In practice, adequate renal function may be assumed to regulate the Cl^-/HCO_3^- balance, and gastrointestinal losses may be replaced litre for litre by 'normal' saline containing 12.5 mmol K^+/l.

ELECTROLYTE AND WATER BALANCE TECHNIQUES

So-called 'fluid balance' is potentially one of the most abused techniques in hospital practice. The routine prescription of a 'fluid balance chart' by the house surgeon presupposes that the keeping of such a balance is of equal importance in all patients for whom it is prescribed and that the nursing staff are able to achieve perfection in all such patients.

It is important to set two standards of accuracy—routine and special:

Routine. Here an accurate record of the *volume and nature of the 24-hour* oral and IV fluid intake, and *24-hour volume of urine* excreted is required:

1. Prescriptions for IV water and electrolyte therapy and for nutrition (p.93) should be arranged in the early morning 06.00–08.00 to achieve consistency of balance studies. Always prescribe each day's IV requirement in legible writing (preferably printing) and on night rounds make sure that the nurse understands it. This eliminates confusion and saves you being woken.

2. When an intravenous infusion fails in the middle of the night, it is only permissible to wait till morning to replace it if the patient is having *maintenance therapy*. When *replacement therapy* is in progress, you must attend to it whatever the hour.

3. Measurement of daily *urine output* by the standard method of measuring and recording each volume passed is adequate. In an adult, provided it exceeds 1 litre daily from the second day after operation, and there are no other excessive losses, the patient may be considered to be in balance.

4. Haematocrit, blood urea, Na^+, K^+, and HCO_3^- concentrations to be estimated every 2 days.

Special. This applies only in complicated cases and must be observed meticulously. *Nothing less than perfection is adequate:*

1. *IV or oral requirements* are prescribed in writing for each 24-hour period. If possible, the patient should be put in a single room so that the traffic of fluid in and out can be more easily controlled. It is best if you personally label the prescribed bottles with the patient's name and number them in sequence. They can be placed by the patient's bed with instructions that none are to be removed, used or unused, until they are checked by you or sister at the end of the period.

2. For each 24-hour period, all *urine* passed is placed without measurement in a container unless, as is frequent, the patient is on an hourly output chart. At the end of the period the 24-hour volume is measured by you or the senior nurse. An *aliquot* is then placed in a specimen bottle and the Na^+ and K^+ measured (and on occasions urea concentration and SG) by the laboratory.

3. All *gastric aspirate*, vomit or other losses are placed in a second container and the volume is also measured at the end of the period and an aliquot sent for Na^+ and K^+ estimation. Laboratories are often reluctant to carry out such determinations. If this is the case standard values can be used to calculate losses.

4. The patient should be *weighed daily* using either an accurate chair balance or a bed-weighing machine. This technique is more honoured in the breach than in the observance, but is extremely useful.

5. Haematocrit, blood urea, serum creatinine, Na^+ and K^+ to be estimated at least twice weekly and the results charted as a graph. Arterial blood pH, P_{CO_2}, base deficit or standard bicarbonate and serum total protein (albumin) may sometimes be required.

INTRAVENOUS FLUID REGIMENS FOR WATER AND ELECTROLYTE REPLACEMENT

It is important to distinguish the three situations in which water and electrolytes are administered intravenously.

Maintenance therapy implies that there are no unusual external losses, and only the normal daily requirements are administered. This is not a strictly accurate description of the immediate postoperative period, for then there may be hidden losses into 'third spaces' such as areas of oedema, but this period will nevertheless be considered under the heading of maintenance.

Replacement of continuing losses is necessary when there is excessive loss from the gastrointestinal or urinary tracts. These losses are often measurable, so the task of replacement is a relatively easy one.

Replacement of past losses is much more difficult, for there is no way of precisely measuring how great these losses have been. A first estimate can be made of their magnitude by a combination of clinical acumen and biochemical measurement, but complete replacement is achieved by successive approximation. A subset of this category is the correction of *acid-base disturbances,* and this topic will be considered separately.

Caloric and (in the *medium term*) nitrogen replacement will also be required and, though it runs hand in hand with water and electrolyte, is more easily considered on its own (p.95).

Maintenance Therapy

The daily maintenance requirements for a resting normal adult in a temperate climate are:

Na^+	90 mmol
K^+	75 mmol
Water	2500 ml

In the perioperative period this prescription is no longer valid (see Table 3) and for very long-term maintenance other cations such as Ca^{++} and Mg^{++} are necessary, as well as a variety of trace elements. Thus we recommend, as a compromise, that a sequence of three maintenance regimens be employed for the first postoperative days; the next 3–5 days; and for the longer-term.

First 1–2 postoperative days. During this time there are two disturbances of water and electrolyte handling which have a bearing on maintenance requirements. On the one hand, the kidney's ability to excrete a water and sodium load is restricted because of the influence of ADH (vasopressin) and aldosterone. On the other hand, there are continuing losses into and around the operative site: damaged capillaries 'leak' a plasma ultrafiltrate into the tissues and serous cavities, and (especially after abdominal operations) there may be sequestration of extracellular fluid into the bowel lumen. The magnitude of both depends on the duration and size of the operation.

An approximate guide to fluid and electrolyte maintenance requirements in the first 1–2 postoperative days is set out in Table 3. It should be emphasised that the regimen takes no account of abnormal external losses, which must be additionally provided for. It should also be emphasised that the regimens assume that there is adequate renal function. After very major operations neither the assumption nor the predictions may be accurate. Thus, it should be noted that on postoperative days 1–5 we have prescribed sodium in excess of the normal daily requirements: this is to allow for concealed losses.

Table 3 Peroperative maintenance regimens (70 kg adult)

Magnitude of Operation	Average Requirements
Minor: hernia, peripheral orthopaedic, uncomplicated appendicectomy	Oral fluids only
Medium: cholecystectomy, vagotomy, hiatus hernia	Peroperative: 1 l Hartmann's Day 1: 1 l Hartmann's, 1 l 5% dextrose Day 2: 1 l Hartmann's, 2 l 5% dextrose + 40 mmol K^+/l
Major: gastrectomy, colectomy, hip replacement	Peroperative: 1 l Hartmann's Day 1: 2 l Hartmann's, 1 l 5% dextrose Day 2: 1 l Hartmann's, 2 l 5% dextrose + 40 mmol K^+/l
Maximal: oesophagectomy, abdomino-perineal resection, open-heart surgery	Peroperative: 2 l Hartmann's Day 1: 2 l Hartmann's 1 l 5% dextrose Day 2: 1 l Hartmann's 2 l 5% dextrose + 40 mmol K^+/l

Postoperative days 3–5. During this period it can be anticipated that the sequestered water and electrolytes will be progressively released, and so be available for redistribution in the extracellular space or for excretion. At the same time the ability of the kidney to excrete a salt and water load returns towards normal, so that there is a greater safety margin.

In the previous 2 days the patient has been provided with adequate Na^+ and water (and indeed is likely to be in positive balance). K^+ intake has been low, but there will have been release of K^+ from cells. Thus up to a deadline of the end of the fifth postoperative day we advise the daily maintenance intravenous intake be:

1 1 Hartmann's solution
2 1 5% dextrose

The 5 day deadline must be a strict one: either the patient is then able to manage a normal oral intake, or intravenous feeding by way of a central venous catheter must be considered. When the total weight loss of the patient, including both preoperative and postoperative weight loss, exceeds or is expected to exceed 10 kg and there is no immediate prospect or oral feeding beginning, then most clinicians agree that intravenous nutrition should be started.

Postoperative day 6 onwards. If continued intravenous maintenance is required it should be by central venous catheter and include nutritional maintenance. The patient is by now in negative K^+ (though this is mitigated if K^+ is included in postoperative maintenance), nitrogen and energy balance, and this must not be allowed to continue. Details of intravenous nutrition are given on p.95.

Replacement Therapy

In addition to the maintenance requirements described above, external losses through drains, fistulae, gastric aspirate or vomitus must be replaced. These are susceptible to accurate volume measurement, so that in the short term they can be replaced by an equal volume of a solution containing approximately Na^+ 150 mmol/l, K^+ 10 mmol/l. Hartmann's solution has the virtue of being commercially available, but contains only 5 mmol K^+/l. We therefore still prefer to use a composite solution for replacement: 1 1 of 'normal saline' (Na^+ 150 mmol/l) plus 5 ml of 20% KCl (K^+ 12.5 mmol/l).

The postoperative maintenance regimen described caters only for normal postoperative conditions. More complicated circumstances exist but cannot be dealt with in detail. For example: paralytic ileus may cause large volumes of extracellular fluid to be sequestrated in the gut; polyuric or oliguric renal failure may require increased or restricted requirement, and cardiac failure may lead to low sodium replacement. The fundamental of management of these situations is to be as accurate as possible in water and electrolyte balance measurement. The *houseman* is critical to its achievement.

Replacement of Past Losses; Water and Electrolyte Lack

Three classical situations are commonly encountered:

Water Lack

Causes. Reduced intake from any cause; continued loss by urine (as in diabetes insipidus) and insensible routes.

Effects. The body dries out, and the patient has thirst, restlessness, hyperthermia, dry mucous membranes, and oliguria. There is no circulatory disturbance because loss is evenly distributed through the whole body water.

Diagnosis. History of low intake or increased insensible loss; oliguria with high specific gravity; high serum Na^+ and osmolality.

Correction. Water by mouth or intragastric tube; IV 5% dextrose.

Control. Monitor thirst, mucous membranes, urine volume, serum Na^+ and osmolality. In the early postoperative period, antidiuresis may keep urine volume low despite adequate replacement.

Sodium and Water Lack

Causes. Diversion of normal body secretions from the gastrointestinal tract; increased renal losses of sodium and water; increased sensible perspiration; 'anatomical third space'. Remember that the obstructed intestine secretes more sodium and water than it absorbs.

Effects. The loss can be regarded as approximately isotonic with the extracellular space, so the latter shrinks without much tendency for water to be transferred from the intracellular compartment. Thus the patient develops low plasma volume and haemoconcentration, with the corresponding signs of hypovolaemia: hypotension, low CVP, oliguria. If loss has been slow there may have been water replacement and low plasma Na^+. This is *not* characteristic of acute disturbances.

Diagnosis. History of loss by vomiting, diarrhoea, fistula or polyuria, signs of hypovolaemia with empty veins, hypotension, low CVP and oliguria; usually no change in plasma electrolytes (but blood urea concentration is raised).

Correction. Replacement with normal saline or Hartmann's solution. It should be noted, however, that profound prolonged polyuria may result in deficiency of electrolytes other than Na^+, e.g. K^+, Mg^{++}, PO_4^-. There is only rarely a need for their replacement.

Control. Monitor blood pressure, pulse rate, CVP, urine output.

Potassium Lack

Causes. Overt losses from the same causes as for sodium lack; in addition starvation, sodium restriction, and diuretics may cause losses of up to 500 mmol K^+ in 10 days, as may rarely a large villous adenoma in the rectum.

Effects. Patient inattentive, weak, depressed and sleepy, adynamic ileus; ECG changes. These may all be exaggerated by accompanying alkalosis (e.g. pyloric stenosis, diuretic therapy). Up to 500 mmol K^+ can be lost without change in serum K^+ concentration.

Diagnosis. From causes and effects. Serum K^+ is a poor guide though low K^+ usually indicates severe depletion.

Treatment. It is usually best to establish urine output of 30–50 ml/h by correcting Na^+ and water depletion before giving K^+. Add no more than 25 mmol K^+ to each litre of fluid except in unusual circumstances. Do not give more than 100 mmol/24 h unless, first, a good urine volume is established and, second, adequate 8-hour control of serum levels can be obtained. Sudden large infusions of K^+ may be extremely dangerous.

Control. Monitor by observation of patient, ECG, and serum K^+. Frequency of observations depends on rate of administration of K^+. However, it should be noted that monitoring serves mainly to detect hyperkalaemia; total body K^+ depletion may be present despite a normal level of serum K^+.

ACID-BASE DISTURBANCES

Of all the aspects of pre- and postoperative management this is one of the most difficult to understand because of the mystique that still surrounds the methods of measurement and the graphical display of results. The houseman will have to learn the particular way in which results are expressed in his own hospital, but the following general guide may be useful in that all other systems can be derived from it.

The body can be looked upon as analogous to a test-tube containing a dilute solution of electrolytes in water. The alveolus is the space above the solution. Increasing or decreasing the partial pressure of CO_2 in the alveolar space increases or decreases the hydrogen ion concentration (strictly speaking 'activity', but the distinction is not important in clinical practice) in the solution because of the equlibrium:

$$CO_2 + H_2O \rightleftarrows H_2CO_3 \rightleftarrows H^+ + HCO_3^-$$

Raising the partial pressure of CO_2 above the solution drives the equation to the right so increasing the H^+ and HCO_3^- concentrations. This is respiratory acidosis. Adding to the H^+ activity in the solution drives the equation to the left lowering CO_2 pressure above the solution (provided there is free escape of the gas). This is metabolic acidosis. Respiratory and metabolic alkalosis are the reverse of these two states.

It is possible to ascertain H^+ activity by measuring pH and to measure PCO_2 directly. From there it is possible to calculate bicarbonate as it is the only 'unknown' in the equation. The three values enable one to see at a glance what the acid-base status is: but a more accurate picture is obtained if a comparison is made between the expected level of bicarbonate for a given H^+ concentration and the *actual* level present. This is the concept of 'standard bicarbonate' and the difference between it and the actual value gives the metabolic component of any particular disturbance. Unfortunately, matters are not made easy by referring to the difference as a 'negative' or 'positive base excess' but most of us eventually come to terms with this.

The various disturbances can be characterised as follows:

Respiratory acidosis	H^+ increased (pH reduced); PCO_2 increased. No negative or positive base excess.
Respiratory alkalosis	H^+ reduced (pH raised); PCO_2 normal or reduced. No negative or positive base excess.
Metabolic acidosis	H^+ increased (pH reduced); PCO_2 decreased.

Metabolic alkalosis H^+ decreased (pH raised); P_{CO_2} normal
or sometimes slightly increased.

Mixed pictures are, needless to say, difficult and can only be diagnosed from the clinical circumstances.

Correction of Disturbances

Respiratory acidosis or alkalosis. Change the pattern of ventilation. Do not use chemical techniques.

Metabolic acidosis. The negative base excess in mmol of bicarbonate multiplied by 15 gives a first approximation to the dose of a 1 mol/ml solution of bicarbonate that should be used. Care must be observed and careful monitoring used.

Metabolic alkalosis. Correction can be accomplished in the same way as for metabolic acidosis but using hydrochloric acid solutions. However, the circumstances in which alkalosis arises in surgical patients in such a way as to require this to be done are rare and complicated (e.g. liver failure), and the acid-base imbalance is best managed by correction of the underlying problem.

'Blood gases'. When a sample is drawn from an artery for pH and P_{CO_2} determinations it is usual to obtain the P_{O_2} value at the same time. This is partly because the association between acid-base disturbance and ventilation is common and partly because the apparatus is designed to give the three answers as a routine. The combined interpretation of pH, and P_{CO_2} and P_{O_2} is considered on p.142.

OLIGURIA AND ANURIA

Oliguria is arbitrarily defined as a urine output of less than 400 ml daily, and anuria a volume of less than 200 ml daily. Either of these may be the result of pre-renal factors (e.g. hypovolaemia); intrinsic renal disease, (e.g. acute tubular necrosis); or post-renal as in obstruction. Absolute anuria (*no* urine) is rare, and usually is caused by obstruction or renal cortical necrosis. It should be noted that acute renal failure, or partial obstruction, may be associated with a normal or increased urine output (polyuric renal failure).

When oliguria or anuria occurs, the following procedure is initiated:

1. *Catheterise* the patient to confirm that there is a disturbance of urine formation, not of flow.

2. Assess *hydration* and *blood volume status.* Consider urinary tract obstruction.

3. Personally measure SG of the first urine available, and arrange or undertake *microscope* examination. SG around 1010 and the presence of red cells, white cells or casts confirms renal damage. SG greater than 1020, in the absence of sugar or protein, suggests that pre-renal factors are responsible.

4. Institute a specially *accurate fluid balance* record.

5. Estimate baseline *haematocrit, blood urea, serum creatinine* and *protein* concentrations, serum Na^+ and K^+. Also estimate *urinary urea* and *creatinine, osmolality* and *electrolytes.* Pre-renal failure is suggested by a low urine Na^+ (less than 20 mmol/l), and a high urine:serum ratio of urea (over 20:1) or creatinine (over 40:1) concentrations. High urine Na^+, or low urine:serum ratios of urea and creatinine suggest intrinsic renal failure.

6. An attempt can be made to provoke an osmotic or pharmacological diuresis to distinguish physiological from pathological oliguria. Before this is done, any blood volume or ECF deficit must be corrected. *Either* 50 ml of 20% mannitol *or* 80 mg frusemide is then given IV over 15 minutes. If frusemide 80 mg has no effect, a larger dose, up to 500 mg IV, may be given once only. In physiological oliguria the resultant urine flow, collected by catheter, should exceed 40 ml/hour.

During or following low blood pressure states frusemide or mannitol may also be given, in an attempt to avert persistent oliguria, after any volume deficit has been corrected.

Management of Established Renal Oliguria or Anuria

General surgical patients can rarely be managed by oral intake techniques. Therefore:

1. The *renal physician* is consulted at the outset.

2. Basic *fluid intake is restricted* to that which covers insensible losses, i.e. 600 ml/24 hours.

3. Additional *water and elelctrolyte* losses are replaced (including those in urine).

4. *Daily* haematocrit, blood urea, serum creatinine, Na^+, K^+, Cl^-, and base deficit or standard bicarbonate are measured.

5. The patient should be *weighed* accurately each day, and should lose 0.2–0.3 kg daily.

Before the blood urea rises above 30 mmol/l, the patient's general condition deteriorates, or the water and electrolyte state becomes seriously unbalanced, dialysis is indicated. In practice, surgical patients are in such a catabolic state that dialysis is usually established early. Early dialysis also allows appropriate nutritional management.

Chapter 9

Nutrition

Many surgical patients suffer from protein energy malnutrition during the course of their illness. This is thought to be significant when more than 15% of body weight has been lost, i.e. 10 kg or more below well weight in the average surgical patient. Although this degree of weight loss indicates that rehabilitation will be prolonged it is not otherwise dangerous unless associated with body protein depletion. A diagnosis of protein depletion can be made when there is evidence of wasted skeletal muscle bellies and also, but not invariably, a low serum albumin. When the value of this is less than 30 g/1 associated dysfunction of many organ systems, particularly the immune system, is common.

NUTRITIONAL ASSESSMENT

When making a diagnosis of significant protein energy malnutrition it is important to remember that it is not the amount of fat and protein that has been lost that matters but how much of these stores remain.

Static nutritional assessment. All patients being admitted for major surgery should have their nutritional state assessed. The aim is to find out how much weight has been lost and what remains of the stores of body fat and protein. Thus a careful history of food intake over the month prior to admission is taken. If only half the normal intake of food has been taken over this time then more than 5 kg of body weight will have been lost. Evidence for increased energy output such as fever, vomiting or diarrhoea should also be sought. After the patient's well weight has been ascertained, he is weighed and the total weight loss is calculated. Fat stores are roughly assessed by palpation of the fat folds overlying the biceps and triceps muscles. Protein stores are similarly estimated by palpating the temporalis, spinati, interossei, biceps and triceps muscles. Serum albumin concentration is measured.

Dynamic nutritional assessment. This is done by weekly measurements of body weight and serum albumin. When the total weight loss exceeds 10 kg (and physical examination confirms that serious erosion of body fat and muscle has occurred) and especially if the plasma albumin level is less than 30 g/l then nutritional treatment is indicated.

When the patient is in the hospital and there is doubt that he is eating properly, it is useful to obtain a dietary analysis by the nursing staff and dietitian acting together to measure and record intake. Though not very accurate in specific terms it can help unmask gross deficiency in intake or provide reassurance that assistance is not needed.

Hidden deficits. It must not be forgotten that starving or semi-starving patients will frequently be short of *water*, have a low extracellular volume because of diminished sodium intake and be short of stores of glycogen and potassium. Replacement of these is indicated before surgery irrespective of more formal nourishment.

INDICATIONS FOR PERIOPERATIVE NUTRITION

Preoperative patients who have evidence of severe weight loss and erosion of protein stores appear to be at increased risk of complications in the postoperative period. It is usual to replete such patients either enterally or parenterally for a 10-14 day period before surgery. Patients who develop a serious postoperative complication (wound dehiscence, intra-abdominal abscess, prolonged ileus) and are not expected to be eating a normal diet during the second postoperative week should always be fed parenterally.

TREATMENT OF PROTEIN ENERGY MALNUTRITION

Requirements. Most general surgical patients will gain body protein and fat with a regimen of no more than 50 kcal kg/body (210 kJ/kg)weight per day at a calorie to nitrogen ratio of 150:1. Many will do so on a lower total energy intake. Fever, burns (which increase heat loss) and sepsis may increase need but these are special circumstances where expert management is needed.

Enteral feeding. Although a skilled dietitian can sometimes improve protein and energy intake in patients in whom the gastrointestinal tract is functioning, the therapeutic result is frequently disappointing. In most patients where nutritional support is indicated and the gastrointestinal tract is functioning, the administration of a defined formula liquid diet through a fine bore nasogastric tube or occasionally a gastrostomy proves to be very satisfactory. The diet is infused continuously day and night and the most satisfactory results are obtained when a volumetric infusion pump is used. It is advisable to introduce the feeding regimen gradually to allow the patient to adapt to it and to minimise side-effects. As a rough guide, 2 litres of half-strength feed can be given in the first 24 hours and the volume and concentration are gradually increased over the following 3 or 4 days until up to 3 litres of the full strength feed is given in 24 hours. This provides 3000 kcal (12.6 MJ) which may be excessive and small elderly female patients can be rehabilitated on little more than half this amount. It is important to monitor patients on enteral feeding daily; this is achieved by recording accurate input and output, daily weight, blood glucose and serum urea, creatinine and electrolytes as indicated.

Nature of the enteral feed. At the last count in the UK there were in excess of 20 different proprietary feeds. The differences between them are mostly minor—calorie nitrogen ratio, fat as medium chain triglyceride and osmolality. For routine use a surgical unit should select a balanced feed and stick to it. Familiarity with one feed is probably the most important factor in success.

Parenteral feeding. Patients requiring nutritional therapy in whom the gastrointestinal tract is *fistulated, blocked, too short, inflamed* or *cannot cope*, will need intravenous nutrition.

1. The nutrient solution. The simplest regimen is a nutrient solution made up in the pharmacy and packaged in a 3-litre plastic bag. The solution contains 1 kcal/ml (4 kJ/ml) and has a calorie to nitrogen ratio of around 150:1. Dextrose provides the energy source and a synthetic amino acid solution the nitrogen source. (See also Table 4.)

Table 4 Composition of 1 litre of standard solution (500 ml 8.5% crystalline amino acid plus 500 ml 50% dextrose)

Volume	1000 ml
Calories	1000 kcal (4.2 MJ)
Dextrose	250 g
Amino acids	42.5 g
Nitrogen	6.25 g
Additions to each unit of base solution (average adult)	
Sodium (chloride and/or acetate, lactate, bicarbonate)	40–50 mmol
Potassium (acetate, lactate, chloride, acid phosphate)	30–40 mmol
Magnesium (sulphate)	2–4 mmol
Phosphate (potassium acid salt)	6–9 mmol
Additions to only one unit daily:	
Vitamin A	5000–10 000 USP units
Vitamin D	500–1000 USP units
Vitamin E	2.5–5.0 i.u.
Vitamin C	250–500 mg
Thiamine	25–50 mg
Riboflavin	5–10 mg
Pyridoxine	7.5–15 mg
Niacin	50–100 mg
Pantothenic acid	12.5–25 mg
Calcium (gluconate)	2.4–4.8 mmol
Optional additions to daily nutrient regimen:	
Vitamin K	5–10 mg
Vitamin B_{12}	10–30 µg Alternatively may
Folic acid	0.5–1.0 mg be given in
Iron	2.0–3.0 mg appropriate
Zinc	1.0–2.0 mg weekly dosages.

Fat emulsions: Half the energy intake may be given in the form of a 10% fat emulsion mixed in with the nutrient solution. Septic patients are easier to manage metabolically when half the caloric requirements are supplied in this way.

Modified formulations may be required for patients with profound protein energy malnutrition (e.g. keeping the sodium intake very low and watching carefully for hypokalaemia), cardiac, renal or hepatic disease; and in the immediate postoperative period.

2. Additives. At the beginning of the course of nutrition the patient should receive:

Vitamin B_{12} 100 μg IM
Folic acid 15 mg IM
Vitamin K 20 mg IM
1 bottle of 20% soybean fat emulsion via a peripheral vein.

The patient may also require administration of:

A soybean fat emulsion weekly to prevent essential fatty acid deficiency
Iron for iron deficiency
Vitamin K, folic acid and vitamin B_{12} if not supplied in the nutrient solution.

3. Delivery. Delivery of the nutrient solution is made directly via a single line through a central catheter. No Y-junction or other entry is permitted to this line which is inviolate. If it is used to measure central venous pressure or for any other purpose it can no longer be used for intravenous nutrition. For this reason all additional fluids are given by separate IV infusions. The catheter is inserted and maintained according to the strict instructions set out on p. 79.

It is usual to administer about half the calculated requirements for the first 1 or 2 days of intravenous nutrition until patient acceptance to the solution is seen. Many complications can be avoided by controlling or correcting cardiovascular instability and metabolic derangements before commencing parenteral feeding.

⌐MPLICATIONS

Sepsis: caused by contamination of solution (rare); or by the administration procedure).

Volume, concentration and compositional imbalances.

Metabolic: hyperglycaemia, hyperchloraemic acidosis, hypophosphataemia, trace element deficiency.

RULES FOR MONITORING

1. Observe all rules for central venous catheters—when in doubt remove catheter and replace the next day.

2. Compute fluid balance daily.

3. Measure body weight daily. If daily increase is greater than 0.3 kg then water is accumulating. If there is a persistent fall in body weight the patient is in negative nitrogen balance.

4. Measure serum sodium, potassium, chloride, phosphate, and glucose daily until patient is stable.

5. Measure liver function tests, Ca^{++}, Mg^{++}, albumin and haemoglobin once weekly.

6. Measure urine glucose concentration every 6 hours or, better, use capillary blood samples 6 hourly to adjust insulin requirements.

7. Carry out a weekly check on all therapy to avoid the all too easy mistake of carrying on a treatment instruction which has become unnecessary.

Chapter 10

Cytotoxic and Immunosuppressive Drugs

SYSTEMIC CYTOTOXIC THERAPY

Despite the relative insensitivity of most solid tumours to chemotherapy, this method of treatment is being used with increasing frequency by surgeons, physicians, radiotherapists and medical oncologists. It is not the role of the house surgeon to determine when they should be used or in what dosage. However, he may be called upon to administer them according to a protocol and he must be aware of their side-effects (see Table 5) and the precautions that should be taken to detect these at an early stage.

Body Weight and Height

These should be measured before each course of therapy because dosage is often based either on body weight or on surface area. The latter is calculated from the *actual* body weight.

Intravenous Administration

Nearly all chemotherapeutic agents are powerful tissue irritants. Therefore they should be administered in as dilute solutions as possible. Large veins on the forearm or in the antecubital fossa may be used but, because of the risk, it is wiser at the outset and when learning to use a vein on the back of the hand or distally in the forearm so that extravasation can be seen quickly and treatment stopped. In order to be certain that the needle is inside the vein, run in normal saline/dextrose before putting the drug into the IV set. Always ask the patient (who may well be drowsy from drugs given to minimise side-effects) repeatedly if the injection is hurting. If extravasation occurs, stop the drip and aspirate back with the syringe. Inject hydrocortisone through the same needle before withdrawal. If need arises, subcutaneous hydrocortisone can also be injected. A cold compress may help and the extravasated area should be dressed well to prevent secondary infection. For long courses of chemotherapy some units use indwelling subclavian catheters and this is recommended.

Table 5 Side-effects of anticancer agents

Drug	Haematological	Gastrointestinal	Dermatological	Other
Actinomycin D	Thrombocytopenia, leucopenia, anaemia.	Anorexia, nausea, vomiting, diarrhoea, proctitis, glossitis, stomatitis.	Alopecia, erythema with desquamation. Acneiform eruption. Hyperpigmentation.	Potentiates radiotherapy.
Adriamycin	Leucopenia, thrombocytopenia, anaemia.	Anorexia, nausea, vomiting, stomatitis, oesophagitis.	Alopecia. Hyperpigmentation.	Cardiotoxic: acute and chronic. Fever. Potentiates radiotherapy. Cumulative dose important.
Bleomycin		Stomatitis.	Dermatitis.	Pulmonary fibrosis. Fever. Cumulative dose important.
Cisplatin		Anorexia, nausea, vomiting, acute diarrhoea. Paralytic ileus.		Highly nephrotoxic. Also audiotoxic, vestibulotoxic, peripheral neuropathy.
Cyclophosphamide	Leucopenia, anaemia, thrombocytopenia.	Anorexia, nausea, vomiting.	Alopecia, hyperpigmentation, ridging of nails.	Haemorrhagic cystitis.
Cytosine arabinoside	Leucopenia, anaemia, thrombocytopenia.	Anorexia, nausea, vomiting.		

Drug	Haematological	Gastrointestinal	Dermatological	Other
DTIC	Leucopenia, thrombocytopenia.	Anorexia, nausea, vomiting. Diarrhoea. 'Flu-like illness.	Alopecia, facial flushing.	
5-Fluorouracil	Leucopenia, thrombocytopenia.	Anorexia, nausea, vomiting. Diarrhoea, stomatitis.	Alopecia.	
Methotrexate	Leucopenia, thrombocytopenia.	Stomatitis, diarrhoea. Hepatic dysfunction.	Alopecia, dermatitis.	Osteoporosis.
Mitomycin C	Leucopenia, thrombocytopenia.	Hepatic dysfunction.		Renal dysfunction.
Mithramycin	Leucopenia, thrombocytopenia, coagulopathy.	Nausea, vomiting. Hepatic dysfunction.		
Nitrosourea	Prolonged leucopenia, thrombocytopenia.	Anorexia, nausea, vomiting.		
Phenylalanine mustard	Prolonged leucopenia, thrombocytopenia.	Anorexia, nausea, vomiting.		
Streptozotocin		Anorexia, nausea, vomiting.		Nephrotoxic.
Thiotepa	Leucopenia, thrombocytopenia.			

Drug	Haematological	Gastrointestinal	Dermatological	Other
Vinblastine	Leucopenia, thrombocytopenia, anaemia.	Anorexia, nausea, vomiting. Stomatitis, constipation or diarrhoea.		
Vincristine		Constipation, abdominal pain.	Alopecia.	Loss of deep tendon reflexes, mild paraesthesiae up to severe peripheral neuropathy. Hoarseness, ptosis, double vision.

Bone Marrow Depression

This is the most constant side-effect. If blood counts are low the dose modification varies according to the agents being used and the protocol being followed, but the absolute granulocyte count and absolute platelet count are the most important for chemotherapy. The house surgeon's role is to make sure that routine blood tests are drawn and any untoward trend reported.

CONTROL OF MALIGNANT PLEURAL EFFUSION

If there is a moderate pleural effusion which is hampering respiration it should be aspirated. A more major effusion should be drained by an intercostal tube. Several agents are used for recurrent pleural effusions. All act as chemical irritants. Some of the agents for this purpose are:

1. Bleomycin,
2. Thiotepa,
3. Mepacrine,
4. *Corynebacterium parvum.*

Before instilling it into the pleural cavity all the fluid should be drained and a tube left in situ. Bleomycin 60–90 mg dissolved in 1–2 ml of 2% lignocaine and diluted in 100 ml of normal saline is instilled into the pleural cavity through a chest drain. The tube is clamped for 4 hours and the position of the patient changed frequently. The local instillation can be repeated for the next 2 days. Side-effects include local pain, fever and loculated pleural effusion. Systemic steroids may be used to reduce the first two of these.

CONTROL OF MALIGNANT ASCITES

The following non-surgical methods are used. Repeated drainage, diuretics, local radiotherapy, cytotoxic agents such as thiotepa, and radioactive colloids such as ^{32}P. The last is not now fashionable because of the danger to staff. Peritoneovenous shunting is commonly used now. Diuretics and a high fluid load (2–3 litres/12 hours) are required to avoid renal failure. Disseminated intravascular coagulation may also rarely occur and pre- and immediate postoperative blood counts (especially platelets) are mandatory.

Chapter 11

Overriding Surgical Emergencies

There are not many situations where seconds or minutes may save or lose a life. Some of these are discussed below. Individually they occur rarely, but one or other may crop up every few months.

CARDIAC ARREST

It is vital that you familiarise yourself with the local instructions regarding the procedure in this situation, which should be posted in every ward and operating theatre, together with an appropriate emergency kit. Similarly, before carrying out any operation, however minor, under general or local anaesthesia you MUST be prepared and able to carry out intermittent cardiac compression.

It is common practice in critically ill patients or in those with 'terminal' disease to make a pre-emptive decision that resuscitation should *not* be attempted. Though distasteful to many, this can both reduce anguish and save scarce resources. The houseman must know the decision for his patients. If he is called elsewhere always assume initially that resuscitation should be undertaken.

Procedure

1. A *single* sharp blow to the precordium may sometimes restore heart action when it is in standstill, but do not rely on it.

The British Heart Foundation Guidelines are excellent in circumstances when the chest is not open and should be followed:

A for Airway. This must be cleared of vomit, obstructions and loose teeth, but not well-fitting dentures.

B for Breathing. If absent, extend the neck, pinch the nose and breathe into the mouth. Two breaths before commencing C.

C for Cardiac compression. By sternal pressure using the heel of hand.

At about 60 beats per minute. If you are on your own, do 2 breaths and 15 cardiac compressions in a cycle. If you have assistance, respiration should be about once every 5 cardiac compressions.

An aggressive attitude to both the speed and force of resuscitating procedures will prove most likely to produce a live patient.

2. *Adequate cardiac pumping* (as judged by a palpable carotid or femoral pulse), with adequate ventilation, will keep the patient's brain oxygenated. **NOW** call for expert help, which may include ECG monitoring, electrical defibrillation, drugs and cardiac pacing. When more expert help is not immediately available it is important to remember that if ventricular fibrillation is suspected, very early defibrillation at 200 joules may be indicated without recourse to an ECG. This must not be regarded as a substitute for cardiac compression.

RESPIRATORY OBSTRUCTION

Causes and Management

1. *Coma.* The commonest cause is the tongue. Nursing the patient on his side with an airway (oropharyngeal but increasingly nasopharyngeal) is important prophylaxis. However, if there is the slightest doubt the patient should be intubated, particularly if he has to be transported either inside the hospital or elsewhere.

2. *After operations* on the neck such as carotid endarterectomy or thyroidectomy. The usual cause is haematoma but occasionally laryngeal oedema may follow extensive dissection. If obstruction is severe and seems progressive, the wound must be opened in the ward but fortunately this is rarely necessary.

3. *Trauma*

(a) *Jaw fractures* and soft tissue injuries—insertion of the finger into the mouth and traction to bring the jaw forward may relieve obstruction. Beware the *broken denture* as an obstructing agent. The same rules apply as for the comatose patient (see above).

(b) *Neck laceration* involving trachea, as in suicidal cut throat. The tracheal fistula can usually be employed as an adequate temporary airway.

4. *Foreign body impacted in larynx.* This is one of the rare situations where if a laryngoscope and the necessary skill to use it are not immediately available, *immediate tracheostomy* may save life.

Where upper respiratory obstruction is increasing, and where the local circumstances permit, *endotracheal intubation* should be carried out. It is the responsibility of every doctor to be able to intubate the larynx, and the skill can be easily learned by apprenticing oneself to an anaesthetist and by the use of models which are widely available. Remember that in some of the situations mentioned the larynx may be distorted by external pressure or by injury. If the cause of the obstruction does not permit intubating, at once personally take the patient to the *operating theatre*, while administering high flow oxygen via a face mask. If possible, have an assistant call theatre to prepare for urgent tracheostomy, and alert your senior. Immediate tracheostomy on the ward is rarely wise.

TENSION PNEUMOTHORAX

The chief circumstances in which this occurs are:

1. After injury.

2. In patients on artificial ventilation when the lungs are inflated by a high positive airway pressure—particularly when there is pre-existing emphysema.

3. After percutaneous subclavian vein puncture (often delayed for up to 2 weeks and hazardous in relation to anaesthesia).

4. 'Spontaneously' from rupture of an emphysematous bulla.

Clinical recognition of the condition is vital. There is gross tracheal and cardiac displacement and evidence of substantial pneumothorax (breath sounds can sometimes be audible through a pneumothorax). You should immediately call your senior and obtain the emergency equipment for inserting an underwater seal drain. Do not attempt endotracheal intubation which is useless and can be positively dangerous. If the patient's condition is *rapidly deteriorating*, immediate decompression of the pleural cavity must be performed by inserting a wide bore needle, even in the temporary absence of tubing and drainage bottle. In more leisurely circumstances inject local anaesthetic into the proposed site of insertion and accompany the patient *personally* to the x-ray department for an *urgent chest x-ray*, taking with you the equipment for insertion of the underwater drain.

Nowadays the underwater seal drain equipment usually takes the form of a disposable set, consisting of a wide bore trocar, surrounded by a catheter. After infiltrating the skin and chest wall down to the pleura with local anaesthetic, a nick is made in the skin with a scalpel blade, the catheter and needle inserted into the pleural cavity, the trocar withdrawn and the catheter connected to an underwater seal drain (or, as a temporary measure, to a one-way valve). Care must be taken not to injure the lung with this trocar and it is always preferable, given time, to carry the incision down to the pleura so that insertion can be under direct vision. The preferred sites for insertion of the catheter are the fourth and fifth intercostal space in the mid-axillary line, or the second interspace anteriorly.

A patient with a pneumothorax must not be anaesthetised without first inserting a chest drain, lest a non-tension pneumothorax is converted into a tension one.

EXTRADURAL HAEMORRHAGE

Where there is a rapid progression of signs suggesting this condition in a patient with a head injury you should:

1. Ensure the patient has an adequate airway, preferably by endotracheal intubation, and there are facilities for artificial ventilation (at least a double-ended airway).

2. Notify the neurosurgeon on call and/or the surgeon in charge of the patient.

3. Alert the neurosurgical theatre staff, if asked to do so.

4. Alert the anaesthetist on call.

5. Make sure facilities for a head shave are available.

6. Take blood for urgent cross-matching of 2 units.

EXTERNAL HAEMORRHAGE FROM A MAJOR ARTERY

It is scarcely necessary to say that the bleeding should be controlled by continued direct pressure, using a hand and swab, and that *you personally* should continue with this until help arrives. Direct clamping of a major vessel is very rarely indicated but clipping a 'spurter' in the scalp can be useful ahead of definitive treatment.

ORDERING PRIORITIES

One of the recurring problems with severely ill or accident patients is ordering priorities so that the important things for immediate management and thus survival are done *at once*. There is always a tendency for x-rays to be taken because of the possible future medicolegal significance or because the casualty officer quite rightly does not want to be castigated for missing something, when what the patient needs is urgent transfer to the operating theatre for control of bleeding, or relief of obstruction. Nursing and administrative staff may become preoccupied with getting details of little significance about the patient or carrying out routine matters such as washing and undressing, when what is wanted is urgent resuscitation, anaesthesia, and definitive treatment of the wounds. Constant thought and attention is needed by all (not least the houseman) to make sure that everyone is continually and constructively busy in the way most suited to the patient's most important problems. We are not suggesting that corners be cut, only that a realistic analysis is made of priorities. As a guide consider the following list of priorities:*

Immediate Priority

Airway.
Mechanisms of respiration.
Arrest of massive bleeding and restoration of blood volume.

Urgent

Relief of cerebral compression by craniotomy.
Assisted respiration if relief of obstruction and/or correction of embarrassed mechanisms has proved ineffective.

High Priority

Relief of severe pain by administering a narcotic analgesic (p.25, but not without consultation in a patient with head injury, respiratory inadequacy or hypovolaemia).

Laparotomy and less commonly thoracotomy for internal injuries (on occasion this may be required more urgently to establish the conditions under which resuscitation may proceed).

Exploration of damaged major blood vessels and/or expanding haematoma.

*From Hamilton Bailey's Emergency Surgery Ed. H.A.F. Dudley, John Wright, Bristol 1986.

Exploration of pelvis and injuries to bladder, urethra, female genitalia.

Relief of constricting limb burns.

Decompression of fascial compartments.

Fixation of fractures if highly unstable or associated with blood vessel or nerve injury.

Less Urgent

Fracture of long bones without the above (however, if there is a need for anaesthesia for other reasons, the fractures should if possible be definitively treated at the same time).

Minimal Priority

Minor fractures of limbs or trunk, minor lacerations and small burns.

Chapter 12

Severe Trauma

Trauma is the commonest cause of death under the age of 40 and causes considerable disability among survivors. In the UK and Australasia, most severe trauma is the consequence of blunt injuries caused by motor vehicle accidents and falls, and to a lesser extent by blows and assaults. However, though still relatively infrequent, penetrating injuries from stabs and gunshot wounds are increasing, especially in urban areas.

PRINCIPLES IN MANAGEMENT

It is worth reiterating that in severe trauma, as in any emergency, diagnosis and treatment must go together. There is not time for taking detailed case histories, making exhaustive examinations and carrying out baseline investigations which have no immediate relevance. Emergency care and resuscitation must often be started forthwith (see also ordering of priorities p. 108). The most common problems requiring care at once are coma, breathing difficulty and shock. The presence of any one of these means, by definition, that the trauma is severe. In any such case the same basic principles apply.

1. Emergency assessment. Before anything else recognise and treat:

    (a) airway obstruction—noisy breathing; no breathing (silence). In obstruction there is often paradoxical movement as well as respiratory distress

    (b) breathing difficulty—tachypnoea; mental confusion; cyanosis; abnormal breathing patterns. These are usually the consequence of chest wall injury (multiple rib fractures) and/or pulmonary contusion and early ventilatory support may be necessary to stabilise the patient both for respiratory function and circulation

    (c) circulatory failure—hypovolaemic shock with cold peripheries, delayed capillary refilling, low arterial blood pressure and rapid weak pulse

(d) cardiac tamponade—arterial hypotension, high jugular and central venous pressure, pulsus paradoxicus. (For airway obstruction see p. 105; tension pneumothorax see p. 106; control of bleeding see p. 107).

2. *Even if the respiratory system is normal* give oxygen to any patient with an injury equal to or more severe than a fractured femur because in such circumstances mild or moderate hypoxaemia is common.

3. *Cross-match blood urgently* (see p. 71). Six units are usually necessary in the first instance. When drawing blood for this purpose try not to forget that an extra 20 ml can be used for baseline determinations: full blood count, urea and electrolytes, liver function tests and where abdominal injury is suspected, an amylase concentration. Blood alcohol is often desirable and in some parts of the world mandatory after road accidents.

4. *Set up one or more intravenous lines* using a 14 or 16 gauge intravenous cannula in the upper limbs only. More than one line tends to complicate management but may be necessary in the seriously hypovolaemic patient. In many experienced trauma units a central venous line will also be inserted.

5. *Give analgesia.* Pain contributes to shock and the moment the injuries have been evaluated, an opiate should be given by the intravenous route as described on p. 25.

6. *Insert a urinary catheter* unless ruptured urethra is suspected. Urine output is an important guide to resuscitation.

7. *Evaluate all injuries.*

The above principles are not necessarily followed in the order described. A judgement on each of the points needs to be made for individual patients.

Evaluation of Injuries

With blunt trauma, injuries are often mutiple. The severity of total body injury is related to the number of separate injuries present and to the extent of these. It is easy to miss injuries in an emergency especially when there is one obvious and threatening injury which demands attention. It is important to look systematically at all body regions: head, face, neck, chest, abdomen, spine, pelvis and extremities. Look at the patient's back as well as the front; pay special attention to regions with external lacerations, contusions and abrasions. Vascular and neurological injuries are very easily overlooked so feel the peripheral pulses (remember these may be feeble or absent clinically in a patient in shock or who is very cold from long exposure).

Regional Examination

1. *Head.* Assess level of consciousness. Inspect ears and nose for CSF and blood. Collect neurological information.

2. *Face.* Look for any bleeding into the nose or mouth. If there is facial injury, is there any threat, immediate or later, to the airway? Is the jaw intact?

3. *Spine.* Is there any indication of cord damage? Assume the possibility of cervical spine injury in any patient with a head injury and manage his movement with great care.

4. *Chest.* Fractured ribs should be indentified by palpation. They are not of themselves of any great importance unless they lead to an area of flail chest or damage the underlying lung. Take a moment to listen to the heart so that a baseline is established should a murmur or bruit be heard subsequently.

5. *Abdomen.* A wide variety of injuries can occur in the closed abdomen. The initial examination is directed to establishing whether

(a) there are signs of peritoneal irritation

(b) there is evidence of flank contusion plus or minus flank tenderness, both of which suggest renal injury. If possible obtain a specimen of urine and examine for haematuria.

Frank signs in the abdomen are an indication for exploration. However, there is often doubt and an unconscious patient causes great difficulty. Peritoneal lavage is then undertaken urgently, particularly when there are other injuries which need attention and it is necessary to be sure that an abdominal problem is not present.

6. *Pelvis.* Pelvic fractures may be difficult to detect clinically, again especially so in the unconscious patient. Blood loss may be massive particularly with posterior fractures involving sacroiliac dislocation. Severe displacement anteriorly should heighten the suspicion of ruptured bladder or urethra.

7. *Extremities.* A litre or more of blood may be lost around a

fractured femur. Long bone fractures are more serious in terms of causing shock and in their subsequent management if they are compound, comminuted, displaced or if there is associated nerve or vascular damage. Remember again to check the peripheral pulses and if possible both sensory and motor function.

8. *External.* Contusions may be extensive and serious, contributing disproportionately to tissue damage and blood loss in patients who have jumped or fallen from high places or who have been run over by heavy vehicles. Friction burns are also common in the latter and initially may be underestimated.

The Patient with Shock

The earliest, most constant and reliable signs of shock are seen in the peripheral circulation: the patient who is cold and who feels cold with pale peripheries is in shock until proven otherwise. In trauma the shock is almost always hypovolaemic but remember the possibility of cardiac tamponade or the much rarer possibility of cardiac contusion. If the neck veins are empty the shock is hypovolaemic until proven otherwise (and that is most unlikely).

There are five possible sites of blood loss which can be associated with shock in the trauma patient.

1. *External,* which is often obvious. Remember, however, that lay people will frequently exaggerate the amount of blood lost at the site of an accident.

2. *Major fractures,* either obvious clinically or seen on an x-ray.

3. *Chest.* An x-ray will detect blood in the chest but to be useful for other purposes do not forget that it must be an upright film. A good quality film which is obtained under your personal supervision may show the tell-tale broadening of the mediastinum which indicates the possibility of aortic rupture—another cause of hypovolaemia.

4. *Peritoneal cavity.* As indicated, clinical signs may make this obvious but peritoneal lavage should be performed if hypotension cannot be explained and there is the slightest suspicion of intraperitoneal injury.

5. *Retroperitoneum.* Such bleeding is particularly difficult to evaluate. It should only be inferred when all other sites have been eliminated. It is further suggested by the nature of the injury and

associated bony damage to pelvis or lumbar spine.

A number of the above sites may be combined in the patient with multiple injuries.

Shock with Distended Neck Veins

The possibilities are cardiac tamponade; cardiac contusion; concurrent myocardial infarction; tension pneumothorax. Though it is possible to tap the pericardium, the best treatment for tamponade producing shock is immediate thoracotomy, if necessary in the A and E department. An early ECG—other priorities permitting—will help diagnose contusion and infarction. (For tension pneumothorax see p. 106.)

Volume Replacement in Shock

The main fluid lost in trauma is blood and almost all patients who are hypotensive and/or noticeably vasoconstricted will need blood transfusion. However, because cross-matched blood is not immediately available, other fluids are used until blood is available. These restore blood volume and therefore blood flow even if they do not provide oxygen carrying capacity. Very rarely, uncross-matched group O Rh negative blood is used in the exsanguinated patient (see p. 72) but this is wasteful. Low antibody titre group O Rh positive blood can be administered to men and to women past child-bearing age.

Usually the first fluid given to the trauma patient should be isotonic saline or Hartmann's solution. Because both these fluids leave the circulation rapidly, 2–3 litres may need to be run in over the first few minutes. Litre bags should be used and the giving set should have facilities for applying pressure. SPPS (p. 76), 5% albumin or gelatin (Haemaccel) should be the second line fluids. After 10–30 minutes blood should be available.

All resuscitation fluids have sodium concentrations similar to extracellular fluid; if they do not they are ineffective for resuscitation and it is folly to try to restore the circulation in a shocked patient using dextrose and water in any concentration. Few trauma patients require any other type of fluid in the first day. Recall though that when looking after such patients in subsequent days they may:

(a) have a lot of excess sodium on board which they will have to eliminate over the next few days

(b) require 'free' water in the form of dextrose solutions.

If the patient in hypovolaemic shock does not respond to the above measures it suggests:

(a) blood loss is continuing and must be sought, found and stopped even if this means operating on a desperately ill patient

(b) the extent of the trauma has been underestimated; patients in shock with severe tissue damage have extensive areas of oedema ('third space') which require more extracellular volume replacement than at first appears necessary. These losses continue, though in diminishing amount, for 36–48 hours (just as happens in a burn). Failure to correct may result in renal failure, adult respiratory distress syndrome (p.143), sepsis and multisystem failure

(c) there is some additional factor such as myocardial damage.

Urine Output

Hourly urine output is a useful guide to resuscitation from shock. The absolute minimum acceptable urine output is 0.5 ml/kg per hour (about 35 ml in an average adult). Up to three times this value is more acceptable but attempts to raise the output above this will usually cause inappropriate fluid retention. Diuretics have no place in initial resuscitation: blood flow must be restored to the kidneys before they can work and if blood flow is restored diuretics are rarely indicated.

Pulmonary Oedema in Shock

Though it can result from injudicious fluid administration in elderly patients, pulmonary oedema in the traumatised patient is more likely to be the consequence of aspiration of gastric content, direct chest wall contusion or less commonly the early onset of ARDS (p. 143).

Head Injuries

Serious head injuries are common though urgent cranial surgery is rarely required (see p. 107). Head injury is frequently only one element of a multiple injury and even if it is the most obvious component it is not necessarily the most important. Do not attribute shock to a head injury. Patients in hypovolaemic shock who also have a head injury require exactly the same fluid therapy as those without cranial damage. Maintenance of cerebral perfusion is vital to survival of neurological function in the head-injured patient. Contrary to popular belief, sodium-containing fluids are not inherently dangerous; however, free water should be carefully controlled, as in excess it can lead to hyponatraemia, hypo-osmolality and thus brain swelling. In the absence of shock, fluids should be restricted to 1–1.5 l/day in the adult.

Neurological evaluation. Factors such as hypoxia, shock, alcohol and other drugs all depress consciousness and may worsen neurological signs. Drugs used in treatment, e.g. anaesthetic or muscle relaxant agents, also interfere with assessment but they may be essential for effective management.

Most hospitals have special forms for both initial and continuing assessment and these should be followed. The majority are based on the Glasgow coma scale for overall evaluation of conscious state. The scale is based on three tests:

Test	Response	Score
Eye opening:	Spontaneous	4
	To name	3
	To pain	2
	None	1
Best verbal response:	Oriented	5
	Confused	4
	Inappropriate	3
	Incomprehensible	2
	None	1
Best motor response:	Obeying	6
	Localising	5
	Withdrawal	4
	Abnormal flexion	3
	Extension	2
	None	1

To this general evaluation must be added focal neurological assessment—reflexes, pupillary signs.

Management decisions. The above information and its change with time enable management decisions to be made. A deteriorating level of consciousness or the presence of lateralising motor or pupillary signs are indications for CT scanning or, in dire circumstances, for emergency burr holes. Carotid angiography for localisation is now rarely used because, where it is available, CT scanning is almost always possible. CT scanning should be used liberally in the head-injured patient as its ability to exclude a focal cause for the patient's state can be very helpful in ordering management. However, if there are pressing and urgent indications for surgical treatment in other regions of the body (e.g. laparotomy or thoracotomy) then CT scanning should not delay these procedures.

RADIOLOGY IN THE TRAUMA PATIENT

1. Patients with depressed levels of consciousness, airway problems or an unstable circulation should not be sent to an x-ray department unless it is vital and, if so, must be accompanied by skilled attendants. Far better to x-ray on site even if this (rarely nowadays) results in slightly less good quality of films.

2. Radiology should be selective in the initial stages. It is not necessary to know radiologically about a suspected undisplaced fracture when other matters are more urgent. Only five examinations should be requested as initial procedures in the A and E department:

(a) *Chest.* As is clear from the previous pages this is the only x-ray ever justified in the unresuscitated patient. If a pneumothorax is obviously present and causing respiratory or circulatory disturbance it is not necessary to take a chest x-ray before treating the condition. Have confidence in your clinical assessment and insert a drain; then take an x-ray

(b) *Lateral cervical spine.* Ideally taken in all patients with head injury or multiple injuries as these dangerous fractures are often missed. In a patient with head or facial injuries, assume initially that cervical fracture is present, apply a cervical collar and take a lateral cervical spine x-ray when the patient has been resuscitated.

(c) *Pelvis.* A pelvic fracture that is not clinically obvious can be the site of unexplained blood loss. A dislocated hip can be missed in a patient with multiple injuries, especially if he is unconscious

(d) *'One shot' intravenous urogram.* In suspected severe renal trauma, this is a useful procedure which often avoids a lengthy session in the x-ray department

(e) *Skull views.* These do not often guide immediate management unless there is a depressed fracture (see CT scan p. 57 and also p. 107).

All other x-rays can be deferred until urgent problems are dealt with and an overall management plan has been worked out. Such examinations include:

(a) *Extremities.* Assessment of the radiological extent of a bony injury is not needed unless
(i) there is a vascular or neural injury
(ii) the patient is going directly to the operating room from the A and E department

(b) *Spine.* Below the cervical region (see above) these are seldom indicated in A and E. Clinical examination is more important

(c) *Abdominal films* in the context of trauma are largely useless. The exception is penetrating missile trauma, when lateral and anteroposterior films are essential to help localise foreign bodies

(d) *Angiography* is required only in special circumstances and can be effectively done in no other place than the x-ray department. Aortography is indicated if rupture of the thoracic aorta is suspected and in general this investigation will then take priority over all other injuries except where laparotomy or craniotomy has to be undertaken at once on clinical grounds. Some trauma teams require angiography in all significant penetrating wounds of the neck and in lower limb injuries with obvious vascular involvement. The house surgeon's job in all these circumstances is to mobilise the resources of the x-ray department as rapidly as possible.

Chapter 13

Surgical Infections: Diagnosis and Treatment

GENERAL

Two large groups of infected cases are met with in surgical wards:

1. where the infection is the primary cause of admission
2. where the infection is acquired in hospital (nosocomial).

A great deal of attention is being paid to the problem of infection and cross-infection. It is quite disastrous when a patient acquires a significant wound or other infection which occurs only because he is in hospital. There are certain rules with regard to the management of those with infections:

1. All patients with an infection capable of being disseminated, whether this is a discharging abscess or wound, gross pulmonary or urinary tract sepsis, or open, infected, skin lesions such as chronic leg ulcers or bed sores, *must* be isolated, either in a side room of the ward or, better, in an isolation block. These precautions are especially important if the patient is receiving or has received an antibiotic.

2. Material from the lesion must be sent for bacteriological culture in all cases.

3. Though most surgical infections are bacterial, viral infections may be present in surgical patients and their aftermath (antigenaemia) may also exist. The two common infections are hepatitis B and HIV (formerly called HTLV III—the AIDS virus). Rules for these vary from hospital to hospital but it is generally agreed

    (a) infectivity is low for both
    (b) extra special care must be exercised by all members of the team to avoid inoculation of blood into themselves—so called 'needle stick'
    (c) barrier nursing is justified in patients who are antibody positive for HIV and have open wounds, and for patients who have surgical complications of AIDS
    (d) there is debate about the routine screening of high risk

patients for either hepatitis B or HIV. It is easily done for the first; moral considerations may interfere with the second. Be sure you are familiar with the local rules.

Some General Principles

1. Diagnosis should be as precise as possible, both clinical—i.e. that there really *is* an infection and where it is—and bacteriological. However, in severe spreading infections, though cultures should always be taken, treatment may have to be instigated before a precise diagnosis is available. An urgent Gram stain of infective material (including a stain of blood withdrawn for culture) may be most helpful.

2. Antibiotics will not cure pus though they may sterilise it and surgical drainage with antibiotic cover is usually indicated. In that many infections are not a danger to life, antibiotics can often be withheld.

3. Prolonged courses of antibiotics are not often required. If a spreading infection in soft tissues is not under control within 3–5 days then there is an undrained focus or the wrong agent is being used.

4. Prophylaxis is the most common source of antibiotic abuse even though it has helped a good deal in reducing surgical mortality and morbidity. Guidance on prophylaxis will be found under specific headings throughout this book and is based on carefully controlled studies. With the exception of the prevention of sepsis in implanted prostheses (e.g. heart valves), very short courses should be used.

5. All antibiotics have side-effects and can, on occasions, be lethally toxic. This is an additional reason for caution in their use. Always inquire assiduously about 'allergies and sensitivities'. However, many of these are side-effects.

6. New drugs, particularly if they are variants on established agents, are usually more expensive and are not necessarily better.

7. Close cooperation with bacteriologists is essential—no one knows everything.

SPECIFIC SURGICAL INFECTIONS

Gram-negative Sepsis

This has replaced infections with *Staphylococcus pyogenes* as the commonest life-threatening infection in surgical patients. The reasons are multiple: better survival of the seriously ill; immunocompromised patients and those who are receiving steroids; 'reservoirs' of organisms and the consequent possibilities of cross infection in intensive therapy units and operating rooms.

It is important to remember that though blood cultures are usually positive, i.e. the patient has septicaemia, all the manifestations are possible with a negative blood culture.

1. The microorganisms are usually, in order of frequency, *E. coli; Aerobacter aerogenes; Ps. aeruginosa; Proteus; Bacteroides.*

2. The clinical antecedents are, again in approximate order of frequency: urinary tract manipulation (catheterisation, cytoscopy, prostatic biopsy), severe peritonitis, biliary tract disease or manipulation (cholangitis, exploration common bile duct); burns; prolonged IV infusion.

3. The manifestations are:

   (a) **Mild**—fever, rigors, 'warm hypotension'

   (b) **Severe**—fever, rigors, disorientation, hyperventilation, 'cold hypotension', metabolic acidosis.

In the mild form the patient is normovolaemic and survival rate is high. In the severe form the patient usually has a complex pre-existing surgical condition, is hypovolaemic and the survival rate is low.

4. Management. In all but the very mildest and transient episodes it is essential to carry out the following:

   (a) draw blood for culture at least twice daily until at least two cultures have been reported negative

   (b) establish a central venous line (p. 79) and control replacement with crystalloid or colloid by measuring CVP. Considerable volumes may be needed in, for example, peritonitis. A level of 9 cm of water should be aimed for

   (c) call for urgent help from experts such as interested surgeons, anaesthetists and cardiologists and, if possible, transfer the patient to an intensive therapy unit

   (d) have an electrocardiogram so as to be sure that you are not confusing septicaemia with myocardial infarction

   (e) establish whether or not the patient is acidotic by arterial pH measurement. Correct acidosis if present (p. 88)

   (f) administer a 'best guess' antibiotic or combination of

antibiotics, preferably after consultation with your senior and/or the microbiologist

(h) inotropic agents, such as dopamine, are sometimes indicated, but see (c) above.

Abscesses

The principles of treatment of these are as follows:

1. As already stated, with rare exceptions, whatever the situation, when there is pus it must be let out. Antibiotics will partly or completely sterilise an abscess, but will rarely cure it or the patient. Conversely, adequate drainage renders an antibiotic unnecessary.

2. In certain instances, fluctuation, the classical sign of an abscess, appears late as a result of the quality of the surrounding tissues, e.g. breast, hand, foot and digits, parotid, ischiorectal fossa. In these cases, if there has been inflammation for more than 48 hours, pus may be presumed to be present and the part should be explored forthwith.

3. An abscess should hardly ever be opened under local anaesthesia, if only because exploration is limited. A regional block is sometimes acceptable.

4. In opening any abscess the incision must provide adequate drainage and the abscess cavity must be explored to break down loculi and remove all dead tissue.

5. A swab of the pus must always be sent to the laboratory for culture during the day, or be personally plated-out at night.

6. In any unusual abscess, part of the wall should be sent for histological examination, and thought given to acid fast or fungal culture.

Wound Infection

Wound infection may be present in several forms usually accompanied by pain:

1. Superficial reddening of skin margins ('stitch abscess'). This requires no specific treatment.

2. Abscess formation

(a) subcutaneous—removal of stitches. Usually in a laparotomy this means laying the wound completely open. Anything less is often associated with continuing discharge from a linear pocket between subcutaneous tissues and abdominal wall

(b) deep in the wound or intraperitoneal—formal drainage may be necessary when the abscess points. If non-absorbable sutures have been implanted, they may have to be removed.

3. Spreading infection, often streptococcal, sometimes anaerobic. Antibiotics are essential.

4. Residual intra-abdominal abscess.

5. Infection at vascular suture lines. This should be treated with the utmost respect because it can lead to fatal secondary haemorrhage. Energetic antibiotic treatment is essential. A trickle of blood is a herald of a major haemorrhage. Summon help at once.

Urinary Tract Infection

Primary. Infections can either involve the bladder (cystitis) or bladder and renal parenchyma (pyelonephritis). While bladder infections are symptomatically distressing, it is infections of the renal parenchyma that cause scarring and impaired renal function. The tendency is to treat initial infections with only short courses of antibiotics (24–48 hours). This approach appears to have two advantages: first, it will cure the majority of infections and reduce antibiotic consumption and, second, if the infection persists, it suggests that there is some underlying abnormality and further investigation is warranted.

Secondary. Investigate and treat the underlying disorder.

ANTIBACTERIAL DRUGS

Penicillins

A large drug family with generally low toxicity. There is an enormous theoretical knowledge and practical experience with their use.

Benzylpenicillin (penicillin G, crystalline penicillin). This was the original penicillin, first used clinically in 1941. Still one of the treatments of choice for many infections, e.g. streptococcal cellulitis and impetigo, gonorrhoea, penicillin-sensitive staphylococcal infections, pneumococcal pneumonia (the commonest cause of lobar pneumonia), and alone or as a component of regimens for less common surgical infections such as anaerobic chest disease, clostridial myonecrosis (gas gangrene) and other varieties of clostridial and anaerobic streptococcal cellulitis, tetanus, postoperative synergistic gangrenes (rare) and actinomycosis.

Only used parenterally with adult doses 2.0–12.0 Mu, (usually 2.0–6.0 Mu) (depending on the particular clinical syndrome) given 2–6 hourly. Generally only used IV, though IM if needed. Added 1% lignocaine reduces local pain.

Procaine penicillin. Only given IM. It provides a longer duration of penicillin activity for up to 24 hours. Used as a component of some regimens for gonorrhoea and syphilis and occasionally for patients with penicillin-sensitive infections for whom low concentrations are acceptable, e.g. pneumococcal pneumonia.

Benzathine penicillin. Only given IM. It provides a very prolonged duration of low level penicillin action for about 3 weeks. Given monthly it is the most effective prophylactic regimen for preventing rheumatic fever, but has no surgical uses.

Penicillin V (phenoxymethylpenicillin). Only used orally where a patient has a penicillin-sensitive infection and may reliably be expected to absorb the drug, e.g. streptococcal pharyngitis, impetigo and pneumococcal pneumonia. It is not effective as treatment for gonorrhoea or syphilis, and food markedly impairs its absorption.

Isoxazolyl penicillins (cloxacillin, flucloxacillin and their relatives). These drugs are not significantly broken down by the beta-lactamase enzymes of *Staph. aureus* which confer penicillin resistance and are still considered the drugs of choice for all penicillin-resistant staphylococcal disease. In most places upward of 75% of *Staph. aureus* both in and out of hospital is now resistant to benzylpenicillin. *Strep. pyogenes* is always sensitive to these drugs too. Both cloxacillin and flucloxacillin may be given parenterally or orally. Blood levels of oral flucloxacillin are about twice those of equal weight doses of oral cloxacillin. Dosage regimens are 1.0–12.0 g/day of cloxacillin (usually 1.0–4.0 g) given 4–6 hourly and of flucloxacillin 750 mg–8.0 g/day given 6–8 hourly. Food impairs the absorption of both these drugs. Many pharmacies stock only flucloxacillin.

'Gram-negative' or 'Broad-spectrum' Penicillins

Ampicillin. This drug added significant numbers of gram-negative organisms, in particular *E. coli* and *Haemophilus influenzae,* to the spectrum of benzylpenicillin. It is used orally and parenterally. With the passage of time, increasing resistance has developed among these organisms, e.g. over 50% of *E. coli* and *N. gonorrhoeae* may now be resistant and up to 50% of *H. influenzae,* although geographical variations are enormous and local information is important. The resistance of *E. coli* has unfortunately diminished the previously very useful role ampicillin played in urinary tract infections and surgical abdominal sepsis. Adult dosage is 1.0–12.0 (usually 1.0–4.0) g/day given 4–6 hourly. Its absorption is impaired by food. A rash in association with treatment does not imply cross sensitivity with other penicillins.

Amoxycillin. This drug has an identical microbiological spectrum to ampicillin which includes all benzylpenicillin-sensitive organisms, many gram-negative bacilli and virtually all enterococci. Used orally it results in blood levels about twice those of ampicillin for the same weight dose; thus 500 mg ampicillin q.i.d. is about equivalent to 250 mg amoxycillin t.d.s. Amoxycillin's absorption is little affected by food.

Ampicillin and amoxycillin are still the most commonly prescribed antibiotics both in and out of hospital. Despite the trends in resistance mentioned, they remain useful for acute purulent exacerbations of chronic respiratory disease, acute otitis media, acute sinusitis, bronchopneumonia, gonorrhoea (though resistance is emerging), acute pelvic inflammatory disease and urinary tract infection (if the bacteria are sensitive). Though diarrhoea and rash, in particular, may be troublesome, their widespread and continuing use reflects their low toxicity and high efficacy. In seriously ill patients, however, who may have septicaemia and for whom correct antibacterial selection is critical, it is important to appreciate that they no longer provide adequate cover against gram-negative bacilli.

Carbenicillin, ticarcillin, piperacillin, mezlocillin and azlocillin. These drugs are used less frequently. They add *Pseudomonas aeruginosa* in particular to the spectrum of ampicillin, although overall gram-negative activity is better than ampicillin. Usually only used for proven or strongly suspected pseudomonas disease. All are only given IV: carbenicillin 20–30 g/day, ticarcillin 12–18 g/day and piperacillin 4–16 g/day. The first two contain high Na^+

concentrations (5 mmol/g of drug) which is potentially important in some patients with fluid and electrolyte imbalance. Piperacillin contains only 2 mmol of Na^+/g. They can also cause hypokalaemia and platelet dysfunction. They are expensive.

Cephalosporins

A family of broad spectrum bacterial drugs, chemically related to penicillins. As a result of major pharmacological manipulation to increase their spectrum of gram-negative activity, they are being used more frequently than previously in sick surgical patients. Cephalosporins have three generations which reflects their historical development and their increasingly broad spectrum of gram-negative bacillary activity (see Table 6).

Table 6 Cephalosporins

First generation	Second generation	Third generation
Cephaloridine	Cefuroxime	Cefoperazone (not available in UK)
Cephalothin	Cefamandole	Cefotaxime
Cephalexin *	Cefoxitin	Moxalactam
Cefazolin	Cefaclor *	Ceftriazone
Cephradine *		Ceftazidine

* Oral preparations. Only cephradine has parenteral preparations as well.

First generation drugs (cephalothin being the most familiar) have broad-spectrum gram-positive and negative activity. They act on penicillin sensitive and resistant (beta-lactamase producing) *Staph. aureus,* streptococci (not enterococci) and many gram-negative bacilli, e.g. many *E. coli,* and *Proteus mirabilis* in particular. In most places gram-negative bacilli, including *E. coli,* have recently tended to develop increasing resistance to these drugs. It is this microbiological event which has stimulated the development of second and third generation cephalosporins resistant to the enzymes which break down their first generation relatives. Local resistance patterns of gram-negative organisms should be known before deciding whether any of these cephalosporins, or which of them, might reasonably be used for gram-negative bacillary disease.

Cephalothin dosage is 1.0–8.0 (usually 1.0–4.0) g/day given IV 4–6 hourly. Cefazolin can be given IM with less pain, and 8-hourly, which some regard as advantageous.

Few important gram-negative organisms are resistant to the second generation drugs, though how long this state of affairs will last remains to be seen. Cefuroxime is conveniently administered as 0.75 g 8-hourly IV, and cefamandole as 1.0 g 4–6-hourly IV. Cefoxitin, alone of the second generation cephalosporins, has significant activity against *Bacteroides fragilis,* the commonest anaerobic isolate in surgical abdominal sepsis. This property, allied to its broad-spectrum aerobic gram-negative bacillary activity, makes it satisfactory used alone for surgical abdominal sepsis in a dose of 1.0–2.0 g 6–8 hourly IV. However, it is the most expensive of the second generation drugs.

The third generation cephalosporins have an increased spectrum of gram-negative activity when compared with second generation drugs and, when gram-negative bacteria are sensitive to both second and third generation drugs, they are virtually always more sensitive to the third than the second (e.g. *E. coli* minimum inhibitory concentration to cefuroxime 2.0 mg/ml, and to ceftriaxone 0.5 mg/ml). Their activity is less against gram-positive organisms (in particular *Staph. aureus*) than first generation drugs and all have useful antianaerobic activity. They do not affect faecal streptococci. Although they added *Ps. aeruginosa* to the cephalosporin spectrum of sensitivity, it is clear that, in general, this has been less effective than originally hoped. Ceftazidine, however, has much the best antipseudomonal activity of those most widely marketed and tabulated in Table 6. The third generation cephalosporins are also developing an increasing role in gram-negative bacillary meningitis. They are expensive.

Cephalosporins are relatively non-toxic; cephalothin does however increase the nephrotoxicity of aminoglycosides. Most need dosage reduction only with severe renal impairment but cephaloridine, the first cephalosporin, is in a separate category and is totally contraindicated in renal impairment. The combination of cephalosporin and a loop diuretic (e.g. frusemide) is nephrotoxic. Allergy, diarrhoea and candidiasis may interfere with therapy. Cephalosporins are frequently recommended as alternative therapies for penicillin-allergic patients unless there is a history of anaphylaxis or rapid onset hypersensitivity.

Aminoglycosides

Gentamicin and tobramycin are broad-spectrum drugs (but with no activity against anaerobic organisms or streptococci). For over a decade they have been the mainstay of therapy in seriously ill patients with actual or presumptive gram-negative bacillary sepsis. Nearly all important gram-negative bacilli (*E. coli, Proteus* spp., *Klebsiella* spp., and *Ps. aeruginosa*) remain sensitive. The well-known problems of oto- and nephrotoxicity are minimised by measuring trough levels of drug and altering dosage and frequency if this rises above 2 mg/l (= μg/ml). Peak levels 30–60 minute post doses should be 6–12 mg/l. Careful adjustment of dose is needed in the presence of impaired renal function. Usual dosage is a loading dose of 2 mg and then 5 mg/kg per day given 8 hourly with monitoring of the drug level.

The earlier aminoglycosides (e.g. streptomycin) are rarely used now. Amikacin is a derivative of the earlier kanamycin and is the most resistant member of this family to the aminoglycoside-inactivating enzymes of gram-negative bacilli. It is currently not for widespread use. Netilmicin is another recently marketed aminoglycoside. Do not mix with broad spectrum antibiotics before administration.

Metronidazole (and Tinidazole)

Metronidazole has an extremely broad spectrum against anaerobes, but has no activity against aerobic or microaerophilic organisms. Virtually all *B. fragilis* isolates are sensitive to it. It is now widely used in many parts of the world alone or as a component of regimens for the management of abdominal sepsis, or prophylactically in large bowel surgery. Parenteral dosage is 500 mg 8–12 hourly IV (the latter dose is most often adequate) and is expensive. It is well absorbed orally (400 mg t.d.s. for anaerobic disease) and rectally as suppositories (0.5–1.0 g 8-hourly). Most patients who need the drug can receive it in either of these non-parenteral ways, effectively and relatively cheaply. It is also effective against protozoa, e.g. *Entamoeba histolytica, Giardia lamblia* and *Trichomonas vaginalis*.

Tinidazole is a slightly less nauseating relative which can only be used orally. Its antimicrobial spectrum is identical. Both may give rise to a metallic taste in the mouth and be associated with a 'disulfiram reaction' with alcohol.

Sulphonamides

These were the earliest widely and successfully used antibacterial drugs but the development of resistance by many organisms reduced their usefulness. *E. coli,* the commonest cause of urinary tract infections, has in many places shown a tendency towards increasing sensitivity over recent years, perhaps related to their less frequent use. They are thus still often inexpensive and effective alternatives for urinary tract infections in particular. There are no clinically important differences between them and sulphadimidine is an effective simple sulphonamide to be arbitrarily selected.

Co-trimoxazole

This drug is a fixed combination of sulphamethoxazole and trimethoprim with broad-spectrum gram-positive and negative activity. It is mostly used for acute purulent exacerbations of chronic respiratory disease and for urinary tract infections. Diarrhoea is a not uncommon side-effect and severe skin rashes, ascribed to the sulphonamide component, are seen occasionally. Generally it is used as a 2 tablet (480 mg) b.d. dosage regimen but a parenteral preparation is available which contains large quantities of sodium. There is microbiological and clinical debate about the need for both drugs in this fixed combination.

Trimethoprim

Given the uncertainties of the need for both components of co-trimoxazole, trimethoprim is now marketed alone in many parts of the world for urinary tract infections. A common dose regimen is to take 300 mg nocte for several days, although for bladder infections with sensitive organisms, as with other drugs, single doses or abbreviated courses are very effective.

Chloramphenicol

This is a famous broad-spectrum aerobic and anaerobic agent limited in its use by an unpredictable capacity to cause fatal aplastic anaemia in upwards of 1 in every 20 000 prescriptions. There are no common surgical indications now other than in neurosurgery, other than in neurosurgery, in particular for cerebral abscess and subdural empyema, and even these indications are diminishing with the advent of effective alternatives. It remains the drug of choice in typhoid fever.

Erythromycin

An effective drug for gram-positive coccal disease which also has significant antianaerobic activity. It is used for staphylococcal and streptococcal disease in patients with penicillin allergy. Usually given four times daily orally as 1.0–2.0 g/day, although parenteral preparations are available. The ester, erythromycin estolate, can cause a painful cholestatic hypersensitivity jaundice and should not be used. Erythromycin is the drug of choice for atypical pneumonias caused by *Legionella pneumophila* or *Mycoplasma pneumoniae*.

Lincomycin and Clindamycin

These drugs were initially introduced for staphylococcal disease, and a particular capacity to penetrate bone was claimed, which suggested a special usefulness in osteomyelitis. Though certainly effective, it was never established that they were an improvement on older more conventional regimens. Recognition of their broad spectrum antianaerobic activity resulted in increasing use in the early 1970s until the potentially fatal large bowel disease (pseudomembranous colitis) became linked with their use. Although this disease, caused mostly by toxin producing *Cl. difficile,* has now been seen with almost all antibacterial drugs, and although there are very clear geographical variations in its incidence, this family of drugs has retained limited use in many parts of the world because of this association.

Tetracyclines

These are broad-spectrum antibiotics with aerobic and anaerobic activity, formerly used in surgery for abdominal sepsis. Resistance in both aerobic and anaerobic gram-negative bacilli has diminished their conventional use in this situation. They remain useful drugs for several important and common community infections, e.g.

acute purulent exacerbations of chronic respiratory disease, acute sinusitis and sexually transmitted chlamydial infections. Doxycycline is a widely used tetracycline at a dose of 100 mg given once a day only with food, and it lacks the major deleterious effects of earlier tetracyclines on already compromised renal function. Tetracyclines are in general potentially nephrotoxic. A considerable number of surgical teams use tetracycline at a concentration of 1 mg/ml to wash out the peritoneal cavity.

Nitrofurantoin

This drug is recommended only for bladder infections; it has no antibacterial effect other than when excreted and concentrated in urine. It is cheap and, though nausea is often a problem, low doses of 50 mg q.i.d. are as effective as the earlier more nauseating larger doses advised. The common bacteria, with the exception of enterococci, remain sensitive to it.

Nalidixic Acid and Norfloxacin

Nalidixic acid is a relatively little used urinary antiseptic which has been available for many years. It is only effective in bladder infections and should not be used in patients with renal failure. Recently, new derivatives of this quinolone class of compounds have been developed and the first of these is norfloxacin. It has a very broad spectrum of gram-negative and positive action including *Ps. aeruginosa* and has been found effective in treating urinary tract infections caused by these organisms. Apart from the rarely used indanylcarbenicillin it is the first therapeutically effective oral agent for *Ps. aeruginosa* infections. Dosage is 400 mg b.d.

ANTIFUNGAL AGENTS

Nystatin

This is a useful anticandida drug. Resistance does not develop to it. It is not absorbed from the gastrointestinal tract and is most useful given for oral candidiasis as a suspension 2 hourly, initially held in the mouth and thereafter 4–6 hourly when the disease is controlled. Candida infection of the mouth is a not uncommon sequel to antibiotic therapy.

Amphotericin

This drug is used parenterally for many systemic fungal infections and is nephrotoxic, causes hypokalaemia and is associated with a local chemical thrombophlebitis. Used as lozenges to suck orally it is an alternative to oral nystatin suspension for oral *Candida* infections.

5-Fluoro-Cytosine

This purine analogue (used orally or IV) is occasionally used in combination with amphotericin for some disseminated fungal infections, e.g. candidiasis.

Ketoconazole

This is the first orally effective drug of the imidazole class which includes the topical agents clotrimazole, econazole and miconazole (also used IV occasionally). It is a broad-spectrum antifungal agent with activity against *Candida* species as well as many dermatophytes. It is used at a dose of 200 mg daily with food. Very rarely it has caused hepatic toxicity and, taken long term, it interferes with androgen metabolism.

PROPHYLAXIS

Introduction

The development of wound infection is determined at the time of operation or shortly thereafter by the implantation of organisms into the tissues. The presence of high tissue antibacterial concentrations at the time of operation prevents multiplication and helps elimination of organisms before they reach numbers that make infection, as distinct from contamination, inevitable.

The following principles govern selection:

1. Use prophylaxis where the frequency and the risks of possible infective complications outweigh the risks, costs and usage difficulties of the prophylaxis.

2. Use drugs which are effective against the likely infecting organisms, cheap and non-toxic.

3. Begin the drugs immediately preoperatively and do not continue for more than 24–48 hours at the very most. There are

studies in many situations which show the efficacy of even single preoperative doses.

Specific Recommendations

The following recommendations are relatively cheap and simple, safe and effective. It is likely that individual surgeons in different parts of the world will have differing views in details about this issue and it is sensible to acknowledge this and use locally established and popular regimens where they differ from these. The principles however remain the same worldwide.

Note that cefazolin recommended in these regimens is a first generation cephalosporin and the least painful intramuscular cephalosporin. The addition of 2.0 ml of 1% lignocaine to other cephalosporins makes all of them acceptable IM if this is a preferred mode of administration.

1. *Gastric and duodenal surgery.* Prophylaxis is *not* necessary for operations where the stomach will not be opened or for operations for duodenal ulcer. Prophylaxis should be used for gastric cancer operations and considered for gastric surgery operations. There is *no* need for routine anaerobic or enterococcal cover for these operations.

Suggested regimens

   (a) Cefazolin 1.0 g IM or IV 0.5 hour preop or IV at operation.
   (b) Cefuroxime 0.75 g IM or IV 0.5 hour preop or IV at operation.

2. *Biliary tract surgery.* Prophylaxis is recommended for those over 70 years, those with acute or recent cholecystitis or cholangitis, obstructive jaundice, common duct stones, biliary tract re-operations and all emergency operations. Patients less than 70 years coming to routine cholecystectomy have a low risk of postoperative infection and most would argue they have no need for prophylaxis. There is *no* need for routine anaerobic or enterococcal cover for these operations.

Suggested regimens

As for gastric and duodenal surgery.

3. *Appendicectomy*. There are many regimens which have been studied and are of more or less equal efficacy. Many surgeons recommend an additional one or two postoperative doses.

Suggested regimens

(a) Suspected 'minor' inflammation without perforation: Metronidazole suppository 1.0 g rectally alone 0.5-2 hours preop
(b) Suspected 'serious' inflammation with local peritonitis:
   (i) as for 'minor' inflammation
   (ii) metronidazole suppository 1.0 g rectally 0.5-2 hours preop, plus cefazolin 0.5 g IM or IV 0.5 hour preop or IV at operation
   (iii) metronidazole suppository 1.0 g rectally 0.5-2 hours preop plus cefuroxime 0.75 g IM or IV 0.5 hour preop, or at operation
   (iv) cefoxitin 1.0 g IM or IV alone 0.5 hour preop or at operation
   (v) metronidazole suppository 1.0 g rectally 0.5-2 hours preop plus gentamicin 120 mg IM or IV 0.5 hour preop or IV at operation.

In the face of peritonitis requiring continuing antibiotic therapy use regimens (iii), (iv) or (v) plus local tetracycline lavage.

It is irrational to combine cefoxitin with metronidazole; the particular merit of cefoxitin over other second generation cephalosporins is its activity against *B. fragilis*.

4. *Large bowel surgery*. Use one of the regimens as for appendicectomy.

5. *High lower limb amputations with peripheral vascular disease*. The risk is clostridial myositis. Benzylpenicillin 1.0 Mu IM or IV 0.5 hour preop and continue 6-hourly for 24 hours.

6. *Transurethral resection of the prostate*. Urologists hold differing

opinions on this issue. Some do not use chemoprophylaxis routinely other than for patients with an indwelling preoperative urinary catheter. Select for known infecting pathogen if the operation has to be carried out in the presence of an established urinary tract infection (see p. 196).

Suggested routine regimen

Cefuroxime 0.75 g IM or IV 0.5 hour preop or at operation and continue 8-hourly for 24–48 hours.

7. *Open prostatectomy.* There is debate over the role of prophylaxis for this operation in the absence of documented infection. Most studies show it not to be effective. If operation must proceed in the presence of infection, select for the known infecting pathogen.

8. *Compound fractures.* Never underestimate the value of wound toilet and do not forget appropriate tetanus prophylaxis.

There seem to be two important aspects of antibiotic prophylaxis which may be forgotten in this particular situation.

(a) Drugs should be used as early as possible in order to convey antibiotic to the contaminated or infected site rapidly.

(b) *Staph. aureus* is the pathogen most commonly isolated from these wounds by the time they reach hospital and remains the commonest cause of later infection. We really cannot hope to prevent infection with every organism ever isolated from these wounds. Thus, while the regimens used may vary, the most important issue is the early use of an effective antistaphylococcal drug. The duration of prophylaxis is a difficult question and there are no clear data which really answer it. For many fractures one dose is probably adequate: for a minority of patients with extensive tissue loss it often means many days or even weeks of 'prophylaxis'. Orthopaedic surgeons will have individual views on duration: most support an arbitrary 48 hours.

Suggested regimens

1. Initial parenteral cephalosporin, e.g. cefazolin 1.0 g IM or IV

(do not use second or third generation cephalosporins: although the gram-negative activity is better, the activity against *Staph. aureus* is less good). Give subsequent parenteral (cefazolin) or oral: e.g. (cephalexin) doses if necessary.

2. Initial parenteral dose of cloxacillin (or flucloxacillin) with subsequent oral or parenteral doses if necessary.

3. Regimen 2. plus initial parenteral ampicillin with subsequent oral amoxycillin or parenteral ampicillin doses if necessary.

If there is major tissue destruction or gross soiling, some add benzylpenicillin 1.0 Mu IM or IV 4–6 hourly to regimens 1. *and* 2. to reduce the risk of gas gangrene.

If there is penicillin allergy—compromise. Use a cephalosporin regimen in the first instance but, if the allergy is really a serious one, consider clindamycin, fusidic acid or co-trimoxazole.

Prophylaxis Against Infective Endocarditis

This is an area of debate and it is not suggested that the regimens which follow are the only possibilities. Nevertheless they fulfil certain basic criteria which, in animal models, seem to be important. These are that the initial dose should produce a very high blood level of antibiotic at the time of the procedure and that a lower level of antibiotic activity should be continued for about 12 hours afterwards.

Which cardiac abnormalities?
Use for:
1. Rheumatic and other acquired valvular disease
2. Prosthetic heart valves including heterograft and allograft valves
3. Congenital heart disease: although it is not theoretically required after complete surgical correction of VSD and of coarctation of the aorta, minor associated abnormalities are often present in these conditions and some believe these constitute a risk.
Consider for:
Permanent transvenous pacemakers: there is debate about this.
Not necessary for:
1. Those who have had coronary artery bypass graft surgery
2. Uncomplicated ASD and repaired PDA.

Which procedures?
1. Dental procedures which cause bleeding.
2. Tonsillectomy and adenoidectomy.
3. Complicated child birth.
4. Urinary catheterisation: given the frequency of this procedure and the rarity of enterococcal endocarditis in most places, it is a reasonable compromise to use prophylaxis only at the time of catheter introduction in those with prosthetic valves or haemodynamically important valve disease.
5. Whether to give prophylaxis to patients at risk who are having upper or lower gastrointestinal tract or respiratory tract investigations is debatable. Although bacteraemia occurs in various percentages of patients undergoing these procedures the development of endocarditis is very rare. Those who are conservative would probably use prophylaxis where the effects of the endocarditis, if it should occur, are particularly serious—this means patients with prosthetic valves in particular.
6. There are many other situations where there may be some risk of bacteraemia, e.g. incision of an abscess and surgery through other infected tissues and sinography. Individual decisions will have to be made on the basis of the likely infecting organism, its sensitivities and its known capacity to cause endocarditis. Do not hesitate to ask local experts.

Which antibiotic regimen?
This is similarly an area of great national and international debate. The regimens which follow are designed to give several options. There are no data which prove one is better than another. Parenteral regimens are probably the more secure because the variable of drug absorption from the gut is bypassed. Recent data show that non-compliance with regimens is an important contribution to failure.

Some countries do not have parenteral amoxycillin available. Then it is appropriate to use parenteral ampicillin in the same dose when parenteral amoxycillin is recommended.

1. *Dental, upper airways and upper gastrointestinal tract procedures*
These regimens are designed to prevent *Streptococcus viridans* endocarditis.
   (a) amoxycillin 3.0 g orally 1 hour preop and consider a further

dose 6 hours later

(b) penicillin V 2.0 g orally 1 hour preop fasting, followed by 0.5 g orally 6-hourly, fasting for two further doses

(c) benzylpenicillin 1.0 Mu mixed with procaine penicillin 0.5 Mu IM 0.5 hour preop

(d) erythromycin stearate 1.5 g orally 1.5–2 hours preop fasting and 0.5 g 6-hourly fasting for 24 hours

(e) vancomycin 1.0 g IV run in over 20–30 minutes preop

Note 1. Patients on penicillin prophylaxis for rheumatic fever should receive regimens (c), (d) or (e).

2. Patients with prosthetic valves should have one of the parenteral regimens.

3. IM penicillins can be made less painful by mixing with 2 ml of 1% lignocaine.

2. *Gastrointestinal tract, urinary tract and obstetric/gynaecological procedures*

These regimens are designed to prevent enterococcal endocarditis:

(a) amoxycillin 1.0 g IM 0.5–1 hour preop or IV 0.5 hour preop or at operation, plus gentamicin 120 mg IM 0.5 hour preop or IV 0.5 hour preop or at operation. Consider repeating both drugs or oral amoxycillin 1.0 g at 6 hours

(b) vancomycin 1.0 g IV run in over 20–30 minutes preop plus gentamicin 120 mg IM 0.5–1 hour preop or IV 0.5 hour preop or at operation.

Note At surgery, these regimens for endocarditis prevention 'take precedence' over those generally used for routine postoperative infection prophylaxis. Both are effective regimens for most of these situations. For colon and appendix surgery the addition of metronidazole makes an effective prophylactic regimen against wound infection.

ANTITUBERCULOUS DRUGS

Specialist advice should always be sought.

1. Initial phase treatment with duration of 2–3 months.
Isoniazid 300 mg daily
Rifampicin 450–600 mg (10 mg/kg) daily
Ethambutol 25 mg/kg daily.

2. Continuation treatment for 9–18 months depending on the anatomical site of the tuberculous infection.
Isoniazid plus rifampicin or isoniazid plus ethambutol (15 mg/kg/day).

There are many variations on these basic regimens which depend on drug resistance of the organisms, drug sensitivity of the patient, costs, severity of the infection and its anatomical site. All have important side-effects and should not be prescribed without consultation.

Chapter 14

Important General Postoperative Complications

TEMPERATURE CHARTS AND THEIR INTERPRETATION

Most surgeons and particularly house surgeons, spend a great deal of time looking at temperature charts, yet surprisingly little thought has gone into their analysis. In the repetitive situation of surgery we can distinguish five broad patterns which, while not absolutely diagnostic, are nevertheless strongly suspicious of particular events (see Figure 2).

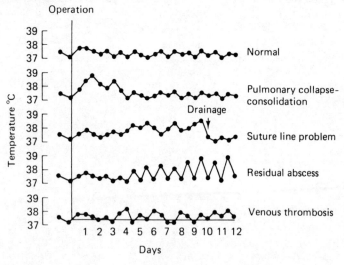

Figure 2

Normal. Even after quite major surgery, provided tissue damage is slight and traumatised tissue is not left in situ, oral temperature rise is small. Two or three readings in the range 37.8–38°C over a period of 24 hours is all that should be expected.

140

Postoperative pulmonary collapse-consolidation with possible super-added infection (see below). This event takes place within an hour or two of leaving the operating table. The effect of retained secretions is an early marked rise in oral temperature to 38.5–38.8°C. Provided that physiotherapy is good and the sputum block eliminated, the fever subsides within 48–72 hours by lysis and the afebrile chart of normal convalescence is resumed.

Suture line dehiscence. It is probable that most suture line problems are the consequence of ischaemia. Therefore as might be expected they begin to manifest themselves at 48–72 hours with a low grade fever which is accumulative over the next approximately 4–5 days. If a drain has been led down to the site of anastomosis then disruption may be followed by fistula formation and lysis of the fever. Otherwise the features of a residual abscess supervene.

Residual abscess. If pus is spilt or organisms introduced at surgery, there is usually a latent period before systemic signs, such as fever, begin to manifest themselves. 72 hours may go by before a swinging chart develops.

Venous thrombosis (see below) when it is spreading is accompanied quite frequently by fever. In that many thromboses begin on the operating table the low grade fever which characterises the condition (37.8–38.8°C) may occur at any time after operation. The diagnosis should be strongly suspected if such a fever persists for 48 hours or more without signs of another complication such as suture line breakdown.

WOUND INFECTIONS

See p. 119.

WOUND DISRUPTION

1. An early warning is the discharge of yellow or blood-stained fluid from the wound, which indicates a peritoneal defect.

2. Delay in the return of bowel function after abdominal operations is occasionally but rarely the result of a gap in the peritoneal suture, allowing a coil of bowel to enter the wound.

3. The skin may gape when sutures are cut out or removed—and there may be underlying deeper disruption not at first obvious.

In all these circumstances the incision is explored and resutured as soon as possible. Inform your senior at once when suspicion arises (before secondary infection has occurred).

Where bowel is visible through a disrupted wound, cover it with a sterile sheet soaked in intravenous saline (*not* cottonwool or similar material), give a sedative premedication, inform your senior and warn the operating theatre and an anaesthetist.

A further episode of frank wound disruption is uncommon (but not unknown): after a first episode consideration should be given to providing supplementary intravenous alimentation (see p. 95) if healing-failure can be attributed to malnutrition. After wound disruption there is a greatly increased incidence of incisional hernia.

RESPIRATORY COMPLICATIONS

Postoperative 'chest' complications are the result of the following sequence of events: hypoventilation (usually the consequence of unrelieved pain), patchy and predominantly basal collapse-consolidation, and finally secondary infections with resident or extraneous organisms. They are thus most likely to occur:

1. When a patient with pre-existing chest disease comes to operation without adequate preparation (p. 31).

2. In abdominal and thoracic surgery where pain-free breathing is most difficult to achieve.

Prophylaxis is by

1. Careful preparation of the patient (p. 32).
2. Ensuring good quality pain relief.
3. Gaining the cooperation of the physiotherapist so that any possibility of sputum retention is minimised.

Mild sputum retention can account for the occurrence of early (first 24 hours) pyrexia in many patients and this should heighten the house surgeon's awareness of the possibility that a chest complication is going to develop. It is only later that classical physical signs—tachypnoea, productive cough and patchy consolidation at the bases—appear. The chest x-ray will show changes from the preoperative film with areas of collapse-consolidation at the bases. Blood gas readings should be obtained on patients with all but the mildest of postoperative chest problems. Note that in the surgical hypoxic patient both the partial pressure of oxygen and that of carbon dioxide are low: the shallow rapid breathing 'blows off' carbon dioxide but, because of the right to left shunt through the collapsed lung, hypoxia persists. Note also that hypoxia can be more dangerous to a surgical patient if areas of the circulation are already ischaemic—such as a recently mobilised skin flap or an intestinal anastomosis.

The treatment of the ordinary postoperative chest problem is largely by physiotherapy unless the patient is severely embarrassed by hypoxia. Quite dramatic improvements can be brought about by vigorous encouragement to cough and for this purpose the patient must be pain free. Oxygen may need to be delivered by face mask but severely compromised patients with cyanosis usually need intubation, tracheal toilet and positive pressure ventilation. Massive bronchial plugging and pulmonary collapse is a rare indication for bronchoscopy.

The place of antibiotics is uncertain. It is best to concentrate on mechanical methods unless the patient is severely systemically disturbed. Sputum cultures should be obtained and organisms such as *Strep. pneumoniae* or *Haemophilus influenzae* treated specifically. Place most emphasis on getting the bronchial tree as clear as possible.

POST-TRAUMATIC PULMONARY INSUFFICIENCY: ADULT RESPIRATORY DISTRESS SYNDROME

After very major injury, but more especially in association with severe sepsis of gram-negative type, patients frequently develop a pulmonary condition characterised by patchy and fluffy consolidation, stiff lungs and severe respiratory insufficiency. The mechanisms are multiple but the effect of bacterial toxins on leucocytes, causing them to marginate in the pulmonary microcirculation and initiate endothelial damage, is probably most important and emphasises the strong association between the condition and sepsis. It tends to creep up on the severely ill patient and vigilance is required particularly in monitoring blood gases. Treatment is in the ITU and largely beyond the scope of this Guide.

DEEP VEIN THROMBOSIS

Prospective studies using research techniques have shown a 30% incidence of thrombosis in the veins of the calf muscles (soleal sinuses) in patients at or beyond middle age who are undergoing major procedures. The incidence of iliofemoral thrombosis either as a primary event or as an extension of calf vein thrombosis is unknown. Clinical trials of *prophylaxis* against calf thrombosis show that conventional early ambulation, lower limb elevation and physiotherapy are all ineffective. Elastic stockings or bandages may have some effect. The following regimens do work:

Heparin.
1. Calcium heparin by subcutaneous injection 5000 units 2 hours before operation, 24 hours postoperation and then twice daily for the duration of confinement to bed
2. Intravenous sodium heparin 1000–5000 units daily.
Dextran 70. 1 litre of 6% solution in normal saline over 6 hours beginning at the induction of anaesthesia.
Calf muscle stimulation and on-table graduated compression. These are specialised techniques and the apparatus is not uniformly available.

Though effective in reducing the incidence of calf thrombosis, none of the above has ever been conclusively shown to prevent pulmonary embolism. However, prophylaxis should be considered in high risk groups which will include one or more of the following characteristics:

1. age over 60
2. obesity
3. malignant disease
4. previous deep vein thrombosis
5. hypercoaguability

It is said that young women on the contraceptive pill are at increased risk but the evidence is scanty. There probably are a few women with an occult hypercoagulability who are in danger but it is extremely difficult to identify them. It is wise to recommend that the pill is stopped at least one month before major elective surgery.

Diagnosis. With a real incidence of calf vein thrombosis of 30%, undetectable in most patients by clinical means, there is no longer any point in routine daily examination of the legs. Nevertheless *low grade fever*, palpable localised *calf tenderness,* or uni- or bilateral ankle *oedema* with increased depth of skin colour or bluish hue, create a high index of suspicion of major deep vein thrombosis. Before potentially dangerous therapy is instituted, objective proof *must* be obtained by phlebography.

The best method of treating deep vein thrombosis is in doubt. A conventional approach is:

1. If signs are confined to the calf, and either Doppler flowmetry or phlebography shows the thrombus is confined to the leg veins, prescribe continuing activity with a firm below knee elastic bandage.

2. If signs are extending or thrombus is detected in the iliofemoral veins by Doppler flowmetry or phlebography, use the same treatment schedule as for pulmonary embolus (see below). Venous thrombectomy in this circumstance has usually not prevented emboli, nor left the patient with a patent vein.

PULMONARY EMBOLISATION

Prospective perfusion/ventilation scanning has shown an 8% incidence of pulmonary embolus in middle-aged surgical patients. The clinically recognised incidence is about 0.5%. There have been no adequately conducted trials that show prophylactic therapy to be effective in reducing the incidence.

The following should create a high index of suspicion that a patient has suffered a moderate sized (e.g. lobar) pulmonary embolus: *breathlessness, pleurisy* (with or without pleural rub), or *haemoptysis.* The following suggest a large pulmonary embolus (blocking at least one main pulmonary artery): *severe breathlessness, faintness, collapse with hypotension, R ventricular heave, gallop rhythm, split pulmonary second sound, elevated R atrial* (jugular venous) *pressure.* Before potentially dangerous therapy is instituted (or continued), objective proof is desirable by *lung perfusion scanning* or by *pulmonary angiography.* Electrocardiographic signs are unreliable, often dangerously so.

The choices of immediate therapy are:

1. *Pulmonary embolectomy* is rarely indicated, requires cardiopulmonary bypass, and demands absolute proof of diagnosis by pulmonary angiography.

2. Fibrinolytic therapy by *streptokinase* or *urokinase* for 24–36

hours followed by heparinisation for at least 7 days. *This is not applicable within 10–14 days of operation.* It is otherwise the most effective therapy (though requiring excellent laboratory control and with significant risk of bleeding episodes).

3. *Anticoagulant therapy.* Intravenous *heparin.* 10 000 i.u. IV stat., then about 1000 i.u./hour by continuous infusion to maintain clotting time at 10–15 minutes; or better, to maintain the activated partial thromboplastin time, kaolin–cephalin clotting time, or thrombin clotting time within the limits recommended by your laboratory.

4. When a *low cardiac output state* is present, and is either immediately life-threatening or does not respond to above therapy, oxygen by face mask or endotracheal tube is administered; inotropic agents are indicated and the patient is transferred to the ITU.

5. When there is proven *recurrence* of pulmonary embolus during or after the above forms of therapy, *inferior vena caval interruption* by ligation, plication, serrated clip, or caval 'umbrella' may be undertaken.

A flow–chart, summarising this information, is shown in Figure 3.

Longer-term therapy, after the initial or recurrent episode has been controlled, is predicated on the risk of continuing pulmonary embolisation. This in turn is dictated by the presence and anatomical location (size) of deep vein thrombi. Every patient who has sustained a pulmonary embolus should undergo *bilateral lower limb phlebography.* If thrombus is detected in the popliteal vein or more proximally we suggest that a 10–14 day course of heparin therapy be followed by a 6 week to 6 month course of oral prothrombin-depressant therapy (phenindione, warfarin). Some authorities suggest an early start to warfarin.

LOW BLOOD PRESSURE STATES AFTER OPERATION

It is often difficult to determine the precise cause of a low blood pressure state, but to do this is of the very greatest importance to the survival of the patient. You must first check that the blood pressure is indeed low: make sure that the sphygmomanometer cuff is properly placed, check auscultatory readings by palpation, try the other arm.

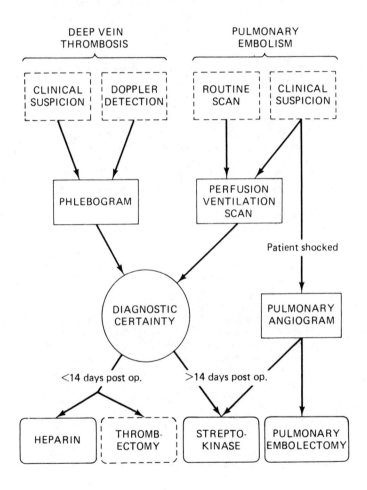

Figure 3

The three major causes of low blood pressure states are:

1. *Reduced blood volume, low cardiac output* = surgical shock. Pallor, sweating, cool extremities, tachycardia, narrow pulse pressure. Consider the possibility of occult bleeding, or pre-existing Na^+ and water depletion. The usual explanation is inadequate replacement of blood previously lost or continuing haemorrhage.

2. *Normal blood volume, normal to high cardiac output* = wide spread arteriolar dilatation. This may occur:

(a) as a consequence of general or regional anaesthesia; of premedicant drugs such as triflupromazine; or of the more specific vasodilator drugs designed to produce hypotension. The patient looks and feels well, and the condition is usually benign: in most instances no more than careful supervision is necessary

(b) as a pre-terminal stage of surgical shock, despite apparently adequate blood-volume replacement; as a result of overwhelming infection (particularly with gram-negative organisms); of the liberation or introduction of gram-negative endotoxins; rarely of genuine adrenal failure. The patient is obviously gravely ill and desperate measures are called for. On the whole it is probably wiser and more profitable to *overtransfuse* with plasma or blood, than to use *vaso-constrictor agents.* Intravenous *hydrocortisone* (250–500 mg) or *prednisone* (50–100 mg) is sometimes dramatically successful, but as a pharmacological agent rather than because of 'adrenal exhaustion'. Where overwhelming infection is suspected, intravenous gentamicin 100 mg or kanamycin 500 mg are probably the most useful antibiotics.

3. *Normal to increased blood volume, low cardiac output* = heart failure—congestive, or specifically right or left-sided. The signs of these conditions should be sought, and the cause: dysrhythmia of sudden onset; pulmonary embolisation; myocardial infarction; K^+ intoxication or gross K^+ depletion; gram-negative septicaemia. *ECG evidence of myocardial infarction should not be too readily accepted*—it is a rare complication in the immediate postoperative period, and the ECG changes may be a result of, rather than a cause of, the low blood pressure.

ACUTE POSTOPERATIVE MENTAL DISTURBANCES

We have already mentioned (p.12) that patients admitted for surgical treatment may be under severe stress and thus behave differently from normal. Sometimes an acute mental disturbance is found in the perioperative period, more usually after operation. When this occurs it is vital to sort out in a logical manner those things that are likely to be the result of an emotional upset and those which are related to physiological or pathological events. In particular it is *never* safe to label a patient as 'mad' or 'having the DTs' just because preoperatively he was known to be a little odd or dependent on alcohol. There are many things such as hypoxia, electrolyte imbalance and severe sepsis, that can mimic delirium tremens in particular and which if not treated early and precisely can lead to the patient's death. The best approach is to run through the following list of causes which is arranged according to frequency and priority in management. If, and only if, no cause is found having gone through this routine is it then justifiable to label the patient as having an acute primary mental disturbance such as a psychosis, and then only after consultation with an enlightened psychiatrist.

1. *Hypoxia.* Obtain and rapidly analyse an arterial blood gas sample. A PaO_2 of less than 50 mmHg should be treated urgently.

2. *Metabolic disturbance.* Hyper- and hypoglycaemia (ward check using a glucose meter); low serum sodium concentration (do electrolyte values); very low or very high serum calcium concentration; low serum magnesium concentration (think of both according to the history and check subsequently).

3. *Sepsis.* Generalised sepsis—syn. septicaemia—draw blood for culture but institute treatment.

4. *Intracranial disorders.* Head injury (fall before or after operation). Cerebral oedema (over infusion).

5. *Situational disorders.* Sleep lack; sensory barrage; inappropriate drugs (check the prescription sheet).

6. *Alcohol.* Delirium tremens (from history of alcohol intake).

Do not make the diagnosis of the last until all others have been excluded. It is one of the **least** common causes.

The treatment of delirium tremens has become much simpler since the introduction of chlormethiazole (heminevrin). It is given as a 0.8% solution initially in an adult at a rate of 5–10 ml/minute. Individual responses vary considerably and it is essential that the patient is carefully observed because he can quickly lapse into deep coma.

POSTOPERATIVE INTESTINAL OBSTRUCTION

Most house surgeons will work in units where they may encounter postoperative disturbances of intestinal function. The basic problem is to distinguish adynamic and discoordinate states (paralytic ileus and pseudo-obstruction) from mechanical obstruction.

Paralytic Ileus

In its true form—complete small and large bowel paresis with no source of mechanical disturbance—the condition is rare. However, the bowel does not function normally for the first 24 hours after major abdominal surgery under general anaesthesia and the colon may take slightly longer to recover, hence the 'windy pains' of which many patients will complain (if asked). However, if a silent abdomen with vomiting or high output from a decompression tube persists beyond 48 hours there is usually something wrong. Principal causes of exogenous paralytic ileus are general peritonitis and residual abscess; retroperitoneal haemorrhage; metabolic disturbance (uraemia, potassium deficiency); ganglion blocking agents.

There is sometimes doubt about whether a patient has ileus after an operation or is vomiting from some other cause. Similarly, after complex surgery it may be quite difficult to tell whether the gastrointestinal tract is ready to accept fluid. The matter can be quite easily settled by the following simple technique which avoids the risk of putting liquid into an atonic receptacle which may result in vomiting.

1. If contrast medium has been used in the preoperative preparation of the patient, take a preliminary portable supine film of the abdomen.
2. Give 50 ml of water-soluble contrast medium by mouth or down the decompression tube.
3. For one hour lay the patient slightly to the right and propped

up so that the medium does not pool in the fundus.

4. Take a further film. Normal progress is diagnosed by finding the contrast medium well down into the distal small bowel. This technique is not designed to give anatomical detail.

Prophylaxis. Obviously all the causes listed should be dealt with. In spite of much work, surgical opinion remains divided about whether decompression of the stomach either by a nasogastric tube or a gastrostomy is helpful in preventing ileus, as distinct from treating it when it occurs. Many surgeons use pre- and postoperative decompression rather sparingly and you must be guided by the local rules.

Management. Any possible cause should be sought and dealt with. Other measures are essentially aimed at maintaining the patient until spontaneous recovery takes place:

1. Gastric decompression.
2. Appropriate fluid replacement—nutrition is required.
3. Remember the 5 day rule.
4. In some intractable cases when everyone's patience is exhausted try pharmacological manipulation:

(a) lay the patient flat and attach a blood pressure cuff to record the arterial pressure on a 5-minute basis

(b) administer intravenously 1 mg guanethidine/minute up to a total of 10 mg. This may itself be followed by loud bowel sounds and a precipitate bowel action but if not

(c) follow straight on with neostigmine 0.1 mg (maximum) up to 1 mg IV

(d) endeavour to make sure before you embark on this regimen that there is either a bed pan or a commode handy and abandon the procedure if there are blood pressure fluctuations.

Mechanical Obstruction

Mechanical obstruction in the first 6 or 7 days after a major abdominal procedure can be difficult to diagnose. It will not often fall to the houseman to make a decision but he should always be on the alert to distinguish paralytic ileus from a real mechanical obstruction. Be particularly vigilant in patients who have had complex surgery, ileostomies or colostomies (where internal hernias are more likely to occur). Bowel sounds and x-rays can both be unhelpful in postoperative patients and only increased distension and 'failure to thrive' may be obvious.

POST-TRAUMATIC GASTRODUODENAL HAEMORRHAGE

It is fortunately fairly rare now for a patient to experience a massive upper gastrointestinal haemorrhage as a consequence of what is generally called a 'stress ulcer' or gastroduodenal 'erosions'. The major determinant is sepsis following in the wake of an acute injury or surgical procedure. The technical management of the incident, if it is allowed to occur, is much as for any other instance of upper gastrointestinal bleeding (p. 186). However, prevention is better than cure. High risk groups include:

1. Major surgery with, or followed by, sepsis as already indicated.
2. Ruptured aortic aneurysm.
3. Burns.
4. Severe head injuries.
5. Massive small bowel resection.
6. Rarely, perforated or bleeding peptic ulcer in which Zollinger-Ellison syndrome (p.45) is suspected.

Two methods of prophylaxis are possible, though the need for either is far from definitely established:

1. If the gastrointestinal tract is intact and functioning, alkalis may be used but have to be in large doses, e.g. 200–300 ml aluminium hydroxide daily in divided doses, or continuously down a nasogastric tube.
2. In other circumstances an H_2 – receptor antagonist 1 g daily by continuous intravenous infusion.

Chapter 15

Abdominal Pain and Acute Appendicitis

One of the commonest reasons for a houseman going to the A and E department is to undertake the initial evaluation of a patient with acute abdominal pain. Though he must always err on the side of caution and consult his senior colleagues before deciding whether a patient should be admitted or sent home, it is worth noting that in most Western communities 30–60% of all patients who present with acute abdominal pain end up with a diagnosis of 'non-specific acute abdominal pain' and that upwards of half of these can have the diagnosis made in the A and E department and not be admitted to hospital.

The causes of acute abdominal pain are legion but, broadly speaking, patients present with pain in either the upper or lower abdomen and the causes correspond. There is overlap, e.g. a perforated duodenal ulcer may produce lower abdominal pain in the right iliac fossa as liquid tracks down the right paracolic gutter, and gonococcal salpingitis can lead to right upper quadrant pain from acute perihepatitis (Fitzhugh Curtis syndrome). However, division into upper and lower is practical in most instances. Patients with upper symptoms and signs are considered under: perforated ulcer, p. 179; acute cholecystitis, p. 170; acute pancreatitis, p. 213. Here we consider central and lower abdominal pain, by far the commonest provisional diagnosis being ?appendicitis.

History

The important points to record are:

1. When the pain started.
2. Where it started.
3. Where it is now.
4. The nature of the pain—constant or intermittent. The pain of appendicitis rarely goes away completely.
5. Loss of appetite, nausea or vomiting.
6. Recent bowel habit—frequency and nature of bowel motions

from 24 hours before onset of pain.
   7. Has there been any urinary frequency?
   8. History of previous similar attacks.
   9. Sore throat or earache in children.
  10. In females:
     (a) menstrual history
     (b) exposure to sexually transmitted disease
     (c) possibility of pregnancy.

Examination

  1. The exact site of maximal abdominal tenderness and guarding.
  2. The presence or absence of a mass. Its size if present.
  3. The presence or absence of rectal tenderness—be sure of the difference between the *discomfort* of the examination and *pain* on digital pressure.

When there is doubt about the diagnosis, the opportunity should be taken to procure a stool specimen for culture and to make sure that there is no blood in the motion.

  4. Vaginal examination should be done in non-virgin females and pain on rocking the cervix sought.

When the diagnosis of appendicitis is unequivocal further investigations are not necessary. In particular, straight x-rays of the abdomen contribute nothing and chest x-rays are only indicated on the usual grounds (p. 61).

However, in a significant number of patients especially young females, uncertainty persists and they are the commonest cause of a negative exploration. The following general rules apply:

  1. Is there urgency or can we observe the patient for 2 hours or so and reassess? Usually the answer is that in the class of patients under consideration there is no hurry (except to get to bed!).
  2. Is pelvic inflammatory disease a possibility? If so some teams would consider laparoscopy.
  3. Is renal tract disease a possibility? Follow the rules on p. 198.

Computers are in use to give a list of probabilities for different diagnoses in the acute abdomen according to the presenting features of individual patients. They have proven their worth in the A and E department. However, their role is mainly to make the houseman collect all the data rigorously. Furthermore, they do not make the diagnosis, they only act as an aid by prompting the clinician.

MANAGEMENT OF APPENDICITIS

Preoperative Preparation

Prophylactic antibiotics should be used in all cases. A standard regimen is metronidazole 500 mg IV or 1 g by suppository (500 mg suppository for children under 12 years of age), plus cephazolin 500 mg IV given with the premedication and followed by two further doses 6 hours apart in the postoperative period.

Appendix Abscess

A localised appendix abscess forms if acute appendicitis is allowed to progress to perforation and the area of inflammation becomes walled off from the general peritoneal cavity. The diagnosis may have been missed or the patient failed to consult a doctor. There is usually a fairly long history of pain (i.e. at least 5 days) and associated pyrexia and leucocytosis.

1. Draw a line on the patient's abdominal wall around the margin of the abscess. Examine daily to assess enlargement or reduction in size.
2. Administer parenteral antibiotics—metronidazole 500 mg IV and cephazolin 500 mg IV 6 hourly.
3. If any of the following develop, surgical intervention to drain the abscess is mandatory:

    (a) enlargement of the mass
    (b) generalised abdominal tenderness indicating peritonitis
    (c) systemic signs of sepsis such as increasing tachycardia or hypotension.

4. Make appropriate investigations after the lesion has settled to exclude carcinoma of the caecum.
5. Interval appendicectomy after 6 months.
Some surgeons will operate on all patients.

POSTOPERATIVE COMPLICATIONS

Peritonitis

If generalised peritonitis is found at operation, make sure a culture of the pus is taken. Delayed primary closure of the wound is advocated (i.e. muscle layer closed but skin and subcutaneous tissues left unsutured and packed). Peritoneal lavage with antibiotics and/or saline will usually have been performed. Antibiotics need not necessarily be continued for longer than the standard two postoperative doses. If delayed primary wound closure has been performed, the skin should be sutured or taped under local anaesthetic 5 days later if the wound is clean. Peritonitis may be associated with septicaemia and blood cultures are routine in the seriously ill.

Abscesses

In most cases of acute appendicitis, even with peritonitis, fever will subside over 2–5 days. If it persists or recurs, suspect:

1. Abscess in or deep to wound—look for reddening, undue tenderness or induration of wound.
2. Pelvic abscess—perform a rectal examination.
3. Subphrenic abscess—examine lung bases, take a chest x-ray (specify the suspected diagnosis so that the radiologist will arrange penetrating views and films on inspiration and expiration).

Vomiting

If this occurs more than 12 hours after operation it suggests a small bowel obstruction on the basis of inflammatory oedema or local or adynamic ileus.

Look for abdominal distension, guarding, absent or obstructive bowel sounds, persistent or increasing fever or tachycardia. Plain x-ray of the abdomen is advisable (see p. 61). When in doubt: start nasogastric aspiration, set up intravenous infusion and inform your senior.

Late Obstruction

Small bowel obstruction may occur later than the eighth day, as a consequence of an abscess or fibrinous adhesions.

A Gastrografin study (see p. 62) may be useful in differentiating mechanical obstruction from ileus. In mechanical obstruction, operation is required.

Chapter 16

Arterial and Venous Surgery

OCCLUSIVE DISEASE OF LIMB ARTERIES

Investigation of patients suspected of this disorder aims at answering in sequence these questions:

1. Is there an *arterial block or stenosis?*
2. *Where* is the block?
3. Are symptoms severe enough, with respect to *pain, work* or *limb survival,* to suggest direct arterial surgery?
4. Does the patient's *general condition* admit of direct surgery, with respect to:
    (a) coronary disease
    (b) cerebrovascular disease
    (c) pulmonary disease
    (d) renal disease
    (e) diabetes mellitus?
5. Is the local arterial condition *technically* amenable to direct surgery?

History

1. *Leg symptoms*
    claudication and walking distance at onset
    rest pain or numbness in the foot
    gangrene
2. *Time relation* of onset of these symptoms.
3. *Site of claudication*
    foot
    calf
    thigh
    buttock
4. Failure of erection.
5. Is the patient incapacitated by his leg symptoms?
6. Symptomatic evidence of disorders affecting his general condition.

Examination

1. *Gangrene* or *foot ulceration,* colour or wasting of limb.
2. Unilateral *skin coldness* of limb and its *upper limit.*
3. *Pulses*—these are most important and must be accurately recorded, as present (+), absent (−), or diminished (±).
4. *Bruits*—listen at carotid bifurcations, *aortic bifurcation* and over *femoral arteries.*
N.B. If a bruit is heard, check that it does not come from *aortic valve* or *aortic coarctation.*
5. Record *blood pressure* in both upper limbs.

General Investigations

Haematology screen, including platelets
Biochemical screen, including serum creatinine and blood glucose
Plasma lipids
Serology for syphilis (not commonly done)
    If a 'collagen' disease is suspected, add:
    ESR
    Serum protein electrophoresis
    Cold agglutinins, cryoproteins
    Antinuclear antibody (or LE cells).
ECG
Chest x-ray

Special Investigations

These depend on the policy and facilities of the unit, but may include indirect measurement of blood pressure at the ankles and direct measurement of femoral artery pressures.

Arteriogram

This is the *last* investigation to be undertaken, if the patient has not already been excluded from surgery. Specify the arteries about which information is sought, and the route suggested by the surgeon for arterial puncture (e.g. 'via right femoral').

Management

If treatment is offered, it is still almost invariably surgical: usually bypass of the arterial occlusion by means of autologous saphenous vein, sometimes endarterectomy. Vasodilator drugs are generally regarded as worthless. Sympathetic ganglionectomy (surgical or chemical) is sometimes used in patients with rest pain when direct arterial surgery is impossible, or as an adjunct to arterial surgery. There is cautious enthusiasm for using balloon dilatation as the first line of treatment in certain arteries (iliacs, renal, coronary) in the case of a short stenosis—that is an isolated lesion.

Specific events to watch for postoperatively are described under Complications.

INTERNAL CAROTID ATHEROSCLEROSIS

History

1. Precise history of *onset* and progress of *neurological episodes*.
2. Historical evidence of *coronary* or *limb atherosclerosis*.

Examination

1. Full *clinical neurological examination*.
2. *Neck*
   common carotid pulses
   external carotid pulses
   (facial, sup. temporal)
   bruit and *site of its maximum intensity but* remember it may occur in absence of atherosclerotic narrowing.
3. Evidence of *limb atherosclerosis* (absent pulses).
4. Fundi for embolic.

General Investigations (As limbs, p.159)

Special Investigations

These may include ocular plethysmography, measurement of the direction of flow in the supraorbital branch of the ophthalmic artery, computerised tomography, dynamic gamma-imaging of the brain (brain scan), and ultrasound imaging of the carotid artery. Unit policy is usually established.

Carotid Arteriography

Only on specific instructions.

Management

Symptomatic lesions are always treated. *Stenoses* are treated by endarterectomy. There is still debate whether very *small lesions,* thought to be a source of platelet or cholesterol emboli, are better treated by endarterectomy or by giving antiplatelet drugs. Asymptomatic lesions (detected with increasing frequency) pose a problem, though most surgeons would recommend endarterectomy for a severe stenosis.

Postoperative care is directed towards the avoidance or urgent correction of hypotension, and the recognition of neurological symptoms or signs. Some surgeons use antiplatelet drugs routinely.

ABDOMINAL ANEURYSM

Leaking abdominal aneurysms present with reasonable frequency to general surgical services.

1. *Suspect* the condition when abdominal pain has been sudden, is severe and unremitting, is also prominent in the back or legs and associated with a fall in BP. Beware the patient with 'left renal colic' who has pallor, tachycardia, and hypotension.

2. *Confirm* the suspicion by allowing the palpating hand to remain on the abdomen long enough to detect the *pulsating mass;* when in doubt, a supine AP and lateral views of the lumbar spine may show calcification in the aneurysm.

3. *Manage* the condition along the following routine lines. The mortality rate is high and the hope of bringing it down lies in being well prepared and able to follow a plan accurately.

4. If the patient is referred from elsewhere:
   (a) obtain as much of the past history as possible
   (b) ask for the most urgent transfer

5. While transport is awaited and/or at the time of admission, as many of the following as possible should be done, but *must not delay* the patient's despatch from elsewhere:
   (a) insert a wide-bore IV cannula into the arm at or above the elbow

(b) blood group: phoning this ahead saves time

(c) draw blood for haemoglobin, creatinine and electrolyte concentrations and phone results when available

(d) insert a self-retaining catheter into the bladder, and measure urine flow

(e) take a lateral x-ray of the abdomen

(f) send all x-rays and notes with the patient

(g) arrange for a doctor to accompany the patient

6. Either at time of referral or if the patient is on your own service at once inform:

(a) surgeon on call

(b) theatre, and ask them to set up a urethral catheter and IV trolley if these have not been done

(c) A & E, particularly to tell them that the patient is to be taken straight from the ambulance to the anaesthetic room

(d) Blood transfusion service to ask for 8 units of blood to be cross-matched

(e) duty anaesthetist

7. When patient is in the anaesthetic room:

(a) reassess: if diagnosis is thought to be incorrect transfer back to the ward; if diagnosis is thought to be established

(b) check efficiency of venous catheter, and establish a CVP or Swan-Ganz line

ARTERIAL EMBOLUS

The situation here has been transformed, so far as limb survival is concerned, by the introduction of Fogarty's embolectomy catheters. Limbs not actually gangrenous can frequently be saved by comparatively simple operations, under local anaesthesia if necessary.

Important practical points are:

1. Whenever a major embolus has possibly occurred, give *heparin* 5000-10 000 u IV *before* detailed investigation: the major cause of failure in embolectomy is propagated thrombus.

2. Though the patient's cardiac state is often poor, major limb or mesenteric gangrene is usually *lethal*.

3. Emboli can be removed from all limb arteries under *local or regional anaesthesia*.

4. In any patient with known mitral stenosis or atrial fibrillation

who develops sudden, severe, abdominal pain—remember *mesenteric embolus.*

5. The commonest complication after embolus is another embolus, so that postoperative anticoagulation may be advisable.

The houseman's role is to recognise the situation and rapidly arrange for surgical intervention.

ARTERIAL INJURIES

1. Arterial occlusion may be caused by blunt injury to the artery from *fracture,* rapid *deceleration,* or near-passage of a *missile.* It may be caused by penetrating injury that *severs* the artery, or that results in a *false aneurysm* which thromboses.

2. Whatever the precise cause, the limb or organ is in immediate jeopardy, with a time limit of *6 hours maximum* before irreversible damage occurs.

3. In any injured patient in whom arterial damage has been possible, *distal pulses* must be sought. If they are impalpable, an arterial occlusion must be assumed and must take *precedence* over all other injuries except those that are immediately life threatening.

RAYNAUD'S PHENOMENON

This term is used to describe a variety of conditions in which some or all of *pallor* or *blueness, pain* and *coldness* occur in the fingers (and sometimes toes). These conditions can be divided into two subsets:

1. Recurrent episodes of a sequence of pallor—blueness—reactive hyperaemia affecting *all fingers of both hands* and associated with cold exposure, lasting minutes rather than hours, and with age of onset usually less than 20 years. This condition is common, often familial, most often affects females, is caused by *cold-induced hyperreactivity* of the digital vessels, and has a uniformly benign prognosis. Occasionally the symptoms result from the use of *vibrating tools* or from *beta-blocking drugs.*

2. An episode of *pallor or blueness* and *severe pain* affecting only *one or a few fingers,* lasting days or weeks, with age of onset usually over 40 years. This is caused by *organic occlusion of digital arteries,* from any one of a wide variety of conditions, the most common of which is *scleroderma.* The outlook is generally bad, with the risk of further episodes and digital tissue loss. Diagnostic tests should be

performed for *scleroderma, blood disorders* including abnormal cryoproteins, and a source of *emboli* should be sought (notably subclavian plaque or aneurysm).

COMPLICATIONS OF ARTERIAL SURGERY

There are many which may occur, but four are of particular importance.

1. *Bleeding.* Postoperative bleeding is easy to detect in the limbs, difficult in the abdomen where it is suggested by falling CVP, falling BP and abdominal swelling. The risk is greatest after surgery for a ruptured aneurysm, or when there has been massive intraoperative blood loss. Treatment by mere blood replacement is not enough: there is either (usually) a blood coagulopathy or (unusually) a technical defect at a suture line.

2. *Sudden occlusion of a graft or prosthesis.* Since the collateral vasculature is usually unprepared, the viability of the distal tissues is often threatened and urgent treatment may be necessary.

3. *False aneurysm,* most commonly at the junction of a prosthesis with the artery and usually the result of a low grade infection. The manifestations may be *fever and local pain;* a palpable *aneurysm;* or *bleeding* from rupture of the aneurysm (including haematemesis and melaena from an aortoduodenal fistula).

4. *Infection.* Apart from the local manifestations of false aneurysm, an infected graft may cause systemic symptoms not unlike subacute bacterial endocarditis.

VARICOSE VEINS

History

1. *Age of onset.*
2. Relation of this to first *pregnancy.*
3. *Number of pregnancies.*
4. Past *superficial venous thrombosis.*
5. Past *frank deep vein thrombosis*—white or blue swollen leg of pregnancy or documented evidence of an episode in relation to severe illness or injury.
6. Past *possible* deep vein thrombosis—? long period of recumbency.
7. *Family history*—did *mother* and *father* have varicose veins?

Examination

1. Skin changes
   eczema
   ulcer
2. Varicose vein distribution
   great saphenous
   small saphenous
   vulval or buttock
   combinations.
3. Is there evidence of sapheno-femoral valvular incompetence?:
   (a) groin thrill or impulse on coughing
   (b) varices controlled by high-thigh tourniquet
   (c) low tension in varices with upright exercise and high-thigh tourniquet.
4. Is there evidence of incompetent valves in perforating veins?:
   (a) dermatofibrosis
   (b) palpable defects in deep fascia (unreliable)
   (c) varices not controlled by mid-thigh tourniquet; and high tension in them with upright exercise and mid-thigh tourniquet.
5. Are ankle pulses absent, suggesting concomitant arterial disease?
6. In an adolescent, are there skin haemangiomas and/or limb overgrowth indicating congenital arteriovenous fistulae?

Special Investigations

The need for these varies from patient to patient and the perception of need varies greatly among surgeons. When there is skin damage caused by valvular incompetence in perforating veins, many surgeons request phlebography to determine if there is stenosis or occlusion of deep, axial veins. If there is access to a vascular laboratory, the surgeon may request dynamic tests (usually Doppler) to determine the presence or location of incompetent perforating veins.

Management

When the main indication for treatment is cosmetic, opinion is divided between surgical treatment, injection sclerotherapy or some combination of the two. When the main problem is skin ulceration, opinion is also divided as to how to treat the underlying venous disorder. Options are elastic support, sclerotherapy, and surgery.

Pre- and Postoperative Care

1. The varices must always be *marked* before operation—usually by the surgeon.

2. After operation there are only two postures permitted the patient:

    (a) *in bed,* with the foot of the bed elevated.
    (b) *actively walking.*

The patient is *not* permitted to sit.

Chapter 17

Biliary Tract Disease

CHOLELITHIASIS

Most patients will be admitted from the waiting list for cholecystectomy and a firm diagnosis should have been made in the outpatients clinic. Review the diagnosis and ensure that all relevant x-rays are available for inspection by the surgeon.

History

It is most important in order to avoid operating for gall stones that are *not* producing the patient's pain, to obtain an accurate history of the exact nature of the acute attacks of pain, with particular regard to its nature; distribution; associated symptoms such as vomiting; and the necessity or otherwise for pain relief. Jaundice must be enquired for, but it must be remembered that a high proportion of patients will state that they become 'yellow' during an attack. It is important to try to obtain objective evidence of jaundice, such as its observation by the general practitioner, or a quite definite association with pale stools and dark urine. Urine colour darkens in most acute illnesses because of a rise in concentration.

The occurrence of fever and rigors must also be enquired for, because they point to cholangitis and to common duct stones.

If there has been a previous biliary operation the patient should be closely questioned about it and if possible full details obtained from the surgeon or hospital concerned: it does not follow that the gall bladder has been removed or all stones removed, even though the patient may think so.

Cholelithiasis is a common condition in countries with a high standard of living, and therefore the radiological demonstration of gall stones may mislead when the pain is caused by some other lesion, e.g. hiatus hernia, peptic ulcer, cardiac ischaemia.

Examination

There are rarely abnormal physical signs referable to gall bladder disease in elective patients and examination is therefore particularly directed at the fitness of the patient for operation.

Investigations

1. Full blood count, creatinine and electrolytes and liver function tests.
2. PA chest x-ray and ECG.
3. Preoperative imaging of the biliary tree—opinions vary but ultrasound is now the commonest.

Preoperative Management

1. All patients who have surgery on the biliary tree should have antibiotic prophylaxis. A suggested regiment is cephazolin 500 mg given intravenously with the premedication followed by two further doses 6 hours apart in the postoperative period.
2. Arrange for an operative cholangiogram.
3. Ensure *all* relevant x-rays are taken to the theatre with the patient.

Postoperative Management

1. Commence oral fluids after 24 hours.
2. Remove the drain after 1–2 days unless there has been significant (100 ml plus) drainage of bile. *Always* check with your senior before drain removal.

3. If a T-tube is in place, this is usually clamped for increasing periods of time from about the fifth day until a T-tube cholangiogram is performed on the seventh day. If clamping produces pain, fever or jaundice this indicates continuing obstruction of the common bile duct. Do not remove the T-tube until the films have been seen by the surgeon.

Postoperative Complications

Bleeding. A moderate amount of blood may be lost through the drain postoperatively, but it is rare for serious bleeding to occur.

Ileus. A mild adynamic ileus often occurs during the first 24 hours after operation. This is rarely of consequence, but if vomiting should persist, abdominal distension occur and bowel sounds not be detectable, bile peritonitis should be suspected. Bile peritonitis is insidious and is often not detected until jaundice from re-absorption becomes obvious.

Pulmonary atelectasis. Followed sometimes by infection, pulmonary atelectasis is a not uncommon complication of cholecystectomy and probably accounts for the fever which frequently occurs in the first 48 hours.

Occult bile leakage. If bile should leak from the site of operation, it may fail to escape from the drain and accumulate first in the subhepatic space and then drain via the right paracolic gutter to the subphrenic space. The effect of this is to rotate the liver downwards to the left and so obstruct the inferior vena cava. The clinical effects are thus often circulatory and the patient may show an insidious onset of circulatory insufficiency which may be confused with a myocardial infarction. Indeed, if myocardial ischaemic changes are already present, they may become intensified as venous return is reduced, thus making ECG interpretation difficult. As long as the possibility of bile accumulation is remembered, early drainage can be instituted.

Retained common duct stones. These may present either as an early complication (filling defects on T-tube cholangiogam) or late complication with jaundice, fever or acute pancreatitis.

Stones may be removed by:

1. Endoscopic sphincterotomy—this has become the procedure of choice (if stone < 2.5 cm in diameter).
2. Burhenne technique—if a T-tube is in place this can be retained for 3–4 weeks until a fibrous track forms. The tube is then removed and a Fogarty catheter or Dormia basket guided into the common duct by a radiologist and the stones retrieved.
3. Dissolution—various substances have been tried such as chenodeoxycholic acid, heparin and mono-octain. These have met with little success.

BILIARY COLIC—ACUTE CHOLECYSTITIS

Common causes of emergency admission are patients with syndromes which range from acute biliary obstruction from a stone impacted in the cystic duct ('biliary colic'), through acute cholecystitis in which a bacterial element may predominate, to acute pancreatitis of biliary origin. The latter probably, but not conclusively, occurs as a result of a stone passing down the common bile duct. The gall bladder in such circumstances is nearly always non-functioning.

History

This is as for non-acute admissions.

Examination

Record:

1. The site of maximal tenderness and guarding.
2. The presence or absence of a gall bladder mass.
3. The presence or absence of jaundice.
4. Fever.
5. Presence or absence of bowel sounds.

Investigations

1. Full blood count, creatinine and electrolytes; liver function tests and serum amylase.
2. Blood culture if fever is present.
3. Biliary excretion scan (^{99m}TcHIDA)—if available, this is the investigation of choice, allowing the diagnosis of acute cholecystitis to be made if there is failure of visualisation of the gall bladder (as a result of cystic duct obstruction) after 60 minutes.
4. Ultrasound—this is the cheapest and most easily deployed method of detecting gall stones and assessing the calibre of intra- and extrahepatic biliary ducts. Its use may be limited because
    (a) it is operator dependent
    (b) gas-filled loops of bowel may obscure the biliary anatomy.

Management

The principal features of treatment in the early stages are:

1. Bed rest, intravenous fluids and analgesia.
2. Antibiotics are not usually indicated.
3. Operation may be performed in the acute phase once the diagnosis of acute cholecystitis has been made. Surgery is usually scheduled for the next operating session but may be performed as an emergency if either systemic disturbances or local signs persist or advance. Acute pancreatitis caused by coexistent biliary tract disease is also an indication for surgery.

Operative treatment is also indicated if there is coexistent cardiorespiratory disease. The risks of surgery are less than those of leaving a large inflammatory mass which impairs ventilation and may embarass the heart because of vasodilatation. Rarely, cholecystostomy may be performed if cholecystectomy is technically impossible. In this case, a cholecystotogram is performed on the seventh day and, if no residual stones are present, the tube is removed. Conventional teaching requires that a cholecystectomy be performed once recovery has taken place. The evidence to support this dogmatic approach is slim.

4. If the acute attack subsides without surgery, biliary tract investigations (ultrasound, IV cholangiogram—though there is debate about the safety of this) are usually performed as outpatient procedures. As there is a risk of further attacks, surgery is carried out as soon as possible after the diagnosis has been made.

OBSTRUCTIVE JAUNDICE

The differential diagnosis usually lies between:

1. Gall stones.
2. Carcinoma—of the head of the pancreas, ampulla, biliary tree (including gall bladder) or metastases in porta hepatis or liver.
3. Cholestasis (drugs, autoimmune hepatitis, rarely viral hepatitis).

When real difficulty exists in the differentiation on clinical grounds, liver function tests are, on the whole, of no further help.

As with many other complex diagnostic problems, a strictly logical approach is useful.

Ultrasound should be the first investigation in obstructive jaundice. If dilated intrahepatic ducts are shown, an extrahepatic obstruction is present and either a percutaneous transhepatic cholangiogram (PTC) or an ERCP should be the next investigation to delineate the level of this obstruction. PTC is now performed with a 'skinny' Chiba needle and the risks of bile leakage are minimal. However, precautions must still be taken to ensure:

1. The patient has a normal clotting profile (prothrombin time and platelet count).

2. Antibiotic prophylaxis is administered—gentamicin 80 mg IV or IM is recommended.

PTC has the advantage that if surgery is not immediately anticipated, the lesion can be intubated with a transhepatic tube at the same procedure to allow biliary drainage. The ease with which these tubes become infected and the detailed care required of them precludes the use of this procedure as a routine preoperative manoeuvre except in specialised units.

Ultimately, if the jaundice is progressively deepening or fails to clear, laparotomy is undertaken. It should be appreciated that the above investigations are not essential prior to laparotomy but only serve to give the surgeon as accurate a picture of the problem as possible. Fortune favours the prepared mind. Operative cholangiography should be arranged.

Special Precautions

Certain special precautions attend laparotomy for jaundice:

1. All jaundiced patients should have a normal prothrombin time (PT) before operation. If the PT is prolonged, vitamin K (10–20 mg IM daily) is given. Measure PT the day prior to operation.

2. Prophylactic antibiotics should be used in all patients. The recommended regimen is: cephazolin 500 mg IV with the premedication and then two further IV doses 6 hours apart in the postoperative period.

Whole gut irrigation (see p. 208) is used by some surgeons preoperatively to reduce the bacterial load in the bowel especially if a biliary-enteric anastomosis is anticipated.

3. Insert a urinary catheter the evening before operation and commence IV fluids to ensure a brisk diuresis before and during surgery (> 60 ml/hour). Mannitol (100 ml of 20% solution) is usually given with the induction of anaesthesia. Careful monitoring of fluid balance and the use of further doses of mannitol or frusemide may be necessary during the postoperative period.

Chapter 18

Breast

ABSCESSES

These present certain difficulties in treatment. They are almost all staphylococcal. The patient will have received some sort of antibiotic therapy before being referred. The abscesses will generally have been present from 1 to 4 weeks and are often *chronic thick-walled abscesses.*

There is a considerable tendency for further loculation of the abscess to occur with imperfect drainage. It is important to ensure that *all* loculi are broken down and all pus and dead tissue removed at the time of initial drainage.

Antibiotics are usually not helpful and should be in any case withheld till culture and antibiotic sensitivity are available. Send the abscess wall for histological examination.

CARCINOMA

The premise usually followed is that all solid lumps in the breast must be submitted to some form of pathological evaluation.

History

Record:
1. Time for which lump has been noticed.
2. Nipple discharge or bleeding.
3. Pain in the breast or the lump and relation, if any, to periods.
4. Lumps which have previously appeared and disappeared.
5. Children and circumstances of breast feeding.
6. Family history of breast cancer.
7. Detailed menstrual history for the last 2 years.
8. Presence of any pain or discomfort elsewhere, particularly bony.

Examination

1. Examination of both breasts, axillae and neck. The *greatest*

diameter of the breast lump, in centimetres, should be recorded. Its position within the breast, and the presence of *any* palpable axillary or supraclavicular lymph nodes should be recorded.

2. Palpable or impalpable liver.

Establishing the Diagnosis

1. Mammography is indicated only to assess the contralateral breast.

2. Fine needle aspiration will

(a) distinguish solid from cystic. Most units do not send breast cyst fluid for cytological examination unless it is blood stained or the lump fails completely to disappear

(b) give a positive diagnosis of malignancy in 80% of patients where it is present. If the houseman does the aspiration he must make three 'passes' through the lesion while applying negative pressure.

3. Needle biopsy is often used particularly in patients where histological confirmation is required before starting non-operative treatment.

4. Open biopsy usually by excision of the lump is now relatively uncommon. Ascertain whether frozen section is needed (again now rare).

Investigations to Find out if Dissemination is Present

In the absence of symptoms:

1. It is usual to defer these until the diagnosis of cancer has been made and appropriate local treatment undertaken.

2. Bone scanning is the most sensitive, but a 'hot spot' should be x-rayed to exclude other bony lesions (e.g. osteoarthritis).

3. Liver function tests are routine in some units but are insensitive.

Assessment of Prognosis and Need for Adjuvant Treatment

1. Oestrogen receptor levels in the tumour cell are increasingly regarded as important. They require 200 mg of fresh tumour preserved in liquid nitrogen until received at the laboratory. When taking such a specimen try to avoid distortion of the specimen (and

particularly the resection margin if a local excision has been used) as this causes unnecessary difficulties for the pathologist.

Preoperative Management

1. Do not use the arm veins on the same side as the lesion for IV infusion or anaesthetic agents. Chronic swelling of the arm and hand is a dreadful complication which may be potentiated by this.

2. Try to ensure that the patient is adequately counselled and comforted before this even more than most operations. A representative of a mastectomy society may be helpful and immediately after that operation arrangements should be made for an external prosthesis.

3. Some treatment options involve radiotherapy or adjuvant therapy. If so, it is best that the radiotherapist and/or oncologist sees the patient before surgery.

Surgical Management

No one standard operation is at all widely accepted, but some form of local excision or mastectomy is likely to be carried out whenever the lesion is locally operable and no distant metastases are evident.

Postoperative Care

Suction drains are now universally used. The tube is removed when the drainage has become minimal, i.e. less than 30 ml daily.

Rehabilitation

Aggressive physiotherapy for early arm movement is unnecessary.

Chapter 19

Burns

There is an increasing tendency to refer burns to special units, where the accumulated experience of the staff can be used to handle the complicated problem of maintaining sterility and replacing damaged skin. Patients with extensive burns travel well in the early stages provided care is taken with fluid and electrolyte management, and with the airway (see respiratory burns below).

In the early phase:

1. Make the distinction between a burn that is possibly survivable and one which is not. This is determined by combining age and extent of burn (disregarding the distinction between deep and superficial). There are tables for this purpose but the matter should be discussed with a senior colleague. It is clearly wrong to expend time and effort to prolong the agony of, say, a patient over 65–69 years with a burn of 68–72% of the body surface; however, every possible effort must be made for a 20–24 year old with the same area as he has at least a 30% chance of survival.

2. Burns over 15% in an adult and over 10% in children (i.e. less than 12 years of age) require intravenous therapy. Establish a line for the administration of fluids early, before hypovolaemia leads to vasoconstriction. Initial resuscitation is with sodium chloride 0.9% or a balanced salt solution, and is guided by observation of peripheral perfusion, pulse, blood pressure, and hourly urine output. The CVP may also be useful.

All patients with burns greater than 25% should have a urinary catheter inserted. The minimum acceptable urine output is 1–2 ml/kg per hour but a greater output is desirable if burns are extensive, as the risk of renal failure is high. Most patients with progressive oliguria in spite of an apparently good circulation will be receiving inadequate fluid resuscitation.

In deep burns, haemoglobin and myoglobin pigments from injured red cells and muscle cells may damage the kidneys and cause renal failure. Patients with extensive burns and darkening urine should have mannitol 1 g/kg body weight and increased fluids to keep ahead of the subsequent diuresis.

3. Determine whether or not there has been a respiratory burn by examining the nose and throat of any patient who has been in a smoke-filled atmosphere or has facial burns. Redness of the fauces or singed hairs in the nostrils warn that oedema of the respiratory tract may develop over the ensuing 12-24 hours. Such a patient should be prophylactically intubated and transferred to a burns unit or failing this to your intensive therapy unit.

Local Treatment

Partial thickness burns—treatment by *exposure* in conditions of low humidity, bacterially-filtered, atmosphere; or by *closed dressings,* using silver sulphadiazine.

Full thickness burns: (a) *very localised*—immediate excision and graft; (b) *more widespread*—treat as for partial thickness burn until about tenth day, when the whole extent of full thickness loss is evident: then split skin graft from patient. If donor skin is inadequate, cadaver allograft or porcine xenograft skin may be used as temporary cover, provided HIV status is determined in the case of allografts.

Chapter 20

Gastroduodenal Surgery

PERFORATED PEPTIC ULCER

History

Enquire for:

1. Convincing history of ulcer pain.
2. Recent exacerbation before perforation.
3. Previous documented proof of an ulcer.
4. Previous or present haematemesis or melaena.
5. Shoulder tip pain.
6. The recent ingestion of drugs which are known to cause gastrointestinal haemorrhage. These include analgesic drugs (e.g. aspirin) and anti-inflammatory agents such as indomethacin and steroids.

Examination

1. A perforated peptic ulcer usually produces generalised abdominal tenderness and guarding with 'board-like' rigidity. Following a perforation high on the lesser curve or in the fundus of the stomach, the signs may be maximal on the left side. Rarely, gastric fluid may leak down the right paracolic gutter and give maximal tenderness and guarding in the right iliac fossa so mimicking acute appendicitis.

2. Percussion to detect the presence or absence of normal liver dullness is important. The replacement of normal liver dullness by a tympanic note is diagnostic of a perforated hollow viscus.

3. Pain may be referred to either shoulder tip but usually to the right as a result of diaphragmatic irritation from gastric contents. This sign can sometimes be elicited by tipping the patient's head down.

4. Assess the patient's general condition, both from the point of view of his present state and of long-standing cardiovascular or respiratory disease.

Investigations

1. Erect PA chest x-ray to detect gas under the diaphragm. Gas beneath the right hemidiaphragm is usually obvious but when present under the left hemidiaphragm it is usually less easily seen. However, if searched for carefully, a thin line of gas can occasionally be seen between the gastric air bubble and the diaphragm in posterior perforations or those high on the lesser curve of the stomach.

Remember that in up to 20% of patients with a perforation, gas will not be seen under either hemidiaphragm.

2. Full blood count, creatinine and electrolytes and baseline blood gases.

3. Group the patients and test for antibodies (see blood transfusion p. 69).

Operative closure of the perforation (usually by suture using an omental patch) and peritoneal lavage should be carried out as soon as the diagnosis is made. Following perforation of a duodenal ulcer, the peritoneal contents are sterile but only for the first few hours. Though many perforations now occur in the elderly as a consequence of anti-inflammatory drugs, with adequate fluid replacement and modern anaesthesia there should nowadays be few indications for non-operative treatment as the risks of sepsis and the non-treatment of a perforated malignant gastric lesion are greater than those of surgery.

For perforation of an acute duodenal ulcer, oversewing with an omental patch is the commonest operation performed. For perforation of a chronic duodenal ulcer, the surgeon usually performs the operation which he routinely uses for elective cases. This may be vagotomy and pyloroplasty, highly selective vagotomy or partial gastrectomy.

If a duodenal ulcer is perforated *and* bleeding, vagotomy and underrunning of the bleeding vessel or a gastrectomy are performed.

For a perforated *gastric* ulcer, treatment is usually gastrectomy. However, if the patient is elderly, the perforation small and peritoneal contamination present, simple excision of the ulcer and closure may be life-saving. The excised ulcer must be sent for histology.

Preoperative Management

1. Morphine or pethidine should be given IM or preferably IV (see p. 25) as soon as the diagnosis has been established.

2. A nasogastric tube may be inserted and the stomach kept empty to reduce further leakage into the peritoneum.

3. An intravenous infusion of crystalloid should be set up.

4. Antibiotic prophylaxis should be given with the premedication. Cephazolin 500 mg IV is recommended. Two further doses are given 6 hours apart in the postoperative period.

Postoperative Management

This is identical to that for elective ulcer surgery below.

Specific postoperative complications:

subphrenic or pelvic abscess

wound infection

pulmonary collapse and/or infection which is particularly a feature of this condition. Vigorous physiotherapy is indicated (p. 142).

Because there is a small possibility of reperforation in the postoperative period (which carries a high mortality), some surgeons believe that intravenous cimetidine should be given until the patient is taking an adequate oral intake.

ELECTIVE ULCER SURGERY

The decision to treat peptic ulcer disease surgically is only taken after serious consideration. Both the choice of patient *and* of operation must be made carefully as poorly planned surgery can lead to failure in terms of recurrent ulcer disease or surgical morbidity.

The main indication for elective ulcer surgery is the failure of the ulcer to heal despite a full course of medical treatment (H_2-receptor antagonists). Surgery may also be advised for the patient whose ulcer has healed but has then recurred, interfering with life and work.

It is vitally important that only patients who will comply with instructions to stop smoking and drinking should be considered for surgery. Selection of patients will usually have been made in the outpatient clinic before admission.

History

1. Total duration of ulcer symptoms.
2. Exact character of pain: situation, radiation, relation to meals, relief by antacids, periodicity.
3. Episodes of haematemesis, melaena or perforation.
4. Vomiting, suggestive of gastric outlet obstruction.
5. The disability suffered by the patient with respect to work, etc. as a consequence of symptoms.
6. Details of past radiological and/or endoscopic diagnosis of peptic ulcer.
7. Details of previous medical or surgical treatment.
8. Particular attention to matters important in the preoperative and postoperative management of the patient, i.e. respiratory or cardiovascular disorders.

Zollinger–Ellison syndrome (ZES), caused by a gastrin-secreting tumour in the pancreas or antrum of the stomach (G cells), is a rare cause of peptic ulcer. In this condition characteristically the ulcer disease is:

(a) aggressive—i.e. has a short history
(b) leads to complications such as haemorrhage and perforation
(c) often multiple
(d) associated with other gastrointestinal symptoms such as diarrhoea.

The proper investigation of any such patient is vital because poorly planned surgery almost always results in a fatal outcome.

Examination

1. Local abdominal signs, particularly localised tenderness suggests activity, as does the presence of a gastric splash or visible gastric peristalsis.
2. Careful examination of cardiovascular and respiratory systems.
3. Examination of the mouth for dental sepsis.

Investigations

1. X-ray chest.
2. Haematology screen.

3. Biochemical screen, including electrolytes, creatinine, and albumin.

4. Have blood cross-matched.

5. Gastric secretory function tests are not used routinely but are indicated when Zollinger–Ellison syndrome is suspected. The features are:

    (a) high resting secretion

    (b) stimulated secretion is only slightly greater than resting.

6. Endoscopy should always have confirmed or reconfirmed the diagnosis before surgery is undertaken.

7. Plasma gastrin levels are measured in:

    (a) suspected ZES.

    (b) recurrent ulcer, especially after gastrectomy.

Preoperative Management

1. If gastric outlet obstruction is present, daily evening stomach washouts with water or saline are performed via a wide bore nasogastric tube. A nasogastric tube should be left in, and nil by mouth ordered. This contracts the stomach and allows easier surgery.

2. An intravenous infusion is set up just before operation.

3. In non-obstructed patients—insertion of a nasogastric tube will normally be performed by the anaesthetist just after anaesthesia is commenced and if requested by the surgeon.

4. Prophylactic antibiotics—a cephalosporin (e.g. cephazolin 500 mg) is given IV with the premedication and again as two further doses 6 hours apart postoperatively.

5. DVT prophylaxis—antiembolic stockings.

6. If a highly selective vagotomy is the planned operation, the surgeon may wish to perform an intraoperative Grassi test in order to 'map out' the acid-secreting region of the stomach. If so, ensure that an ampoule of pentagastrin is sent to theatre with the patient and that a pH meter with a glass electrode is available.

Operative Procedures

The standard procedures practised are:

1. Highly selective vagotomy (HSV)
2. Selective or truncal vagotomy plus:
    (a) pyloroplasty or

(b) antrectomy

3. Partial gastrectomy with gastroduodenal anastomosis (Billroth I)—for gastric ulcer only.

4. Partial gastrectomy with gastrojejunal anastomosis (Polya type).

Postoperative Management

The patient may require intravenous fluids and gastric aspiration for several days, especially after selective or truncal vagotomy. Gastric aspiration should be continuous. Intravenous fluid requirements are discussed in the appropriate section (see p. 84).

Oral fluids are started when the gastric aspirate is less than 200 ml/day, when bowel sounds are present and when the patient has passed flatus. Initially 30 ml/hour are given and the stomach aspirated 4-hourly. The nasogastric tube should be removed as soon as the 4-hourly aspirate is substantially below the oral intake. Since the stomach is readily aspirated by the tube, some surgeons start oral fluids after the first 24 hours. If a gastrostomy is used as a method of draining the stomach, it should be retained until the stomach is firmly sealed to the wall—about 8 days.

GASTRIC CANCER

There is no satisfactory curative, or indeed palliative treatment for this condition other than surgery. From the point of view of cure, the results of surgery are poor. However, as with carcinoma of the large bowel, surgery offers excellent palliation of symptoms, and is undertaken whenever it is thought the patient's general condition permits gastrectomy and whenever it is technically feasible to resect the growth.

History

The important points are:

1. Anorexia may be the first symptom.

2. Enquire about previous dyspeptic symptoms and weight loss.

3. Enquire about previous gastric operations—carcinoma can sometimes arise in a gastric remnant.

Examination

Abdomen. A search should be made for:

1. An upper abdominal mass.

2. Evidence of gastric outlet obstruction in the form of a succussion splash and/or visible peristalsis.

3. The presence or absence of a palpable liver.

Chapter 21

Gastrointestinal Bleeding

MASSIVE UPPER GI TRACT BLEEDING

This is a common cause of hospital admission. The cause varies from place to place but it is most commonly the result of duodenal or gastric ulceration. The patient is often first managed by a medical team but surgeons should be involved from the outset. There is an increasing tendency to undertake joint management. The problem is two-fold:

1. To control the circulatory insufficiency caused by blood volume reduction and often by coexistent cardiopulmonary disorders in elderly patients.
2. To identify the site of bleeding.

In doing the first it is necessary to take into account the very real possibility that an elderly patient may have had a myocardial infarction as a consequence of reduction in blood volume, in which case transfusion necessary to correct anaemia must be cautious.

Upper GI endoscopy as soon as the circulation is stable provides the most accurate way of determining the site of bleeding.

Rarely, for recurrent bleeding of obscure origin, superior mesenteric and coelic angiography may be helpful in locating the source.

Immediate Management

1. Insert a large peripheral line for fluid replacement and a central line for pressure measurement.
2. Cross-match adequate blood (6–8 units). Carry out baseline investigations including liver function tests if varices and/or heavy alcohol intake are suspected.
3. Record an ECG.
4. Arrange an urgent endoscopy.
5. Be prepared to follow on with arrangements for operation or other treatment.

MASSIVE LOWER GI TRACT BLEEDING

Profuse rectal bleeding can present as serious a surgical problem as that of upper GI haemorrhage. Patients are commonly elderly and bleeding usually originates in the colon. Diverticular disease and/or angiodysplasia are responsible for the majority of cases of massive lower GI haemorrhage—colorectal carcinoma never presents with haemodynamically significant rectal bleeding.

Haemorrhage is often severe enough to cause haemodynamic decompensation. In most instances, bleeding will stop spontaneously following blood transfusion but, in some, continued blood loss will necessitate colonic resection.

Rectal bleeding occurring in children is almost invariably caused by haemorrhage from a Meckel's diverticulum and this can be located by a radionuclide scan using technetium-99 pertechnetate.

As for upper GI tract haemorrhage the aims are:

1. To control the circulatory insufficiency by blood transfusion.

2. To identify the site of bleeding—accurate localisation enables a limited colectomy to be performed if bleeding persists.

Immediate Management

1. Cross-match blood (at least 5 units).

2. Carry out baseline investigations.

3. Sigmoidoscopy—usually unhelpful as massive lower GI tract haemorrhage is rarely caused by a local anal or rectal cause.

4. Colonoscopy—when available, this provides one of the most accurate methods of determining the site of bleeding. It may also have a therapeutic role as areas of angiodysplasia can be coagulated. It may be impossible against the tide of blood.

5. Emergency selective arteriography (ESA)—this is the diagnostic investigation of choice in massive lower GI tract haemorrhage providing the exact location of bleeding in up to 80% of cases. Angiography is only of benefit during active bleeding, requiring a blood loss of over 1.0 ml/minute (1440 ml/24 hours). The disadvantages are that it requires an experienced radiologist to perform the investigation and that there is a morbidity attached to femoral catheterisation in elderly patients with arteriosclerotic vessels. A major advantage is that direct embolisation of the bleeding point can be carried out thus reducing the need for surgery

in some cases.

6. Barium enema—is no longer used in the acute situation but to image the colon once bleeding has settled.

The flow chart in Figure 4 gives a guide as to the management pattern.

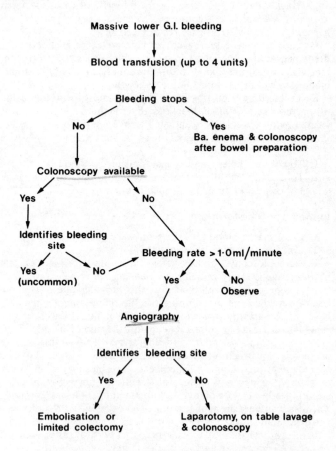

Figure 4

Chapter 22

Genitourinary Surgery

ACUTE URINARY RETENTION IN THE MALE

This is one of the most common urological emergencies and it is most frequently the result of prostatic obstruction in elderly males. However, in any man suspected of having urinary retention it is always important to entertain the possibility of anuria, which can be present even though catheterisation yields up to 300 ml of urine. It is imperative to record the volume of urine in the bladder and to follow output for 6 hours or so after the patient is catheterised so as to avoid confusing a low output with retention.

General Investigation and Initial Management

History. Note the age of the patient. In a male under 50 be cautious in diagnosing prostatic obstruction and consider stricture or a neurological cause. In any patient with urinary retention, ask about the nature of the stream, hesitancy, frequency of micturition by day and night and the ability of the patient to empty his bladder completely. Enquire about haematuria, symptoms suggestive of infection, previous urinary tract surgery, injury or instrumentation of the urethra. A detailed history of bowel function must be obtained. Ask whether the patient has been constipated recently, as constipation can be an important predisposing factor in the development of urinary retention in the elderly male with only minor prostatism. If any doubt exists as to the cause of retention, a careful neurological history must be taken with specific questions about sensory and motor function of upper and lower limbs. Ask about previous back symptoms or injuries. It is also important to obtain information about the cardiorespiratory and central nervous systems for the assessment of the fitness and suitability of the patient for operation.

Examination. A number of special points should be emphasised:

1. A palpable bladder usually confirms the diagnosis of retention.

A tender bladder suggests *acute* retention. A large non-tender bladder with dribbling from the penis (retention with overflow) suggests chronic retention, or may indicate a hypocontractile bladder.

2. The penis must be examined carefully to exclude a tight phimosis or a meatal stricture.

3. Rectal examination. To assess the size of the prostate a variety of reference standards have been used which range from grams to pieces of fruit. The absolute size of the gland is of importance only to the surgeon who is going to perform the operation. The consistency of the gland requires the greatest attention. It is the feel of the gland that usually gives the first hint of carcinoma. Any hard nodule or a hard irregular prostate must be considered to be malignant until proven otherwise. It is important to remember that one is performing a rectal examination and not just feeling the prostate; assess the tone of the anal sphincter, examine the rectal mucosa, seminal vesicles and rectovesical pouch. If the prostate feels malignant, examine carefully for para-aortic and supra-clavicular nodes, liver enlargement and bony tenderness, as the findings may be helpful subsequently in the staging of the carcinoma.

Relief of Retention

The first step in the treatment of most patients with retention is to obtain free bladder drainage, usually by urethral catheterisation.

Though perurethral catheterisation in prostatic obstruction is usually straightforward, occasionally a catheter will not pass. The problem can sometimes be overcome by the passage of sounds and the introduction of a catheter using a Foley introducer, but this approach can have disastrous consequences in inexperienced hands and should *not* be undertaken by a houseman. A false passage can be produced even by a soft catheter and injudicious attempts to pass instruments along the urethra will often only increase the problem. In such circumstances it is preferable to resort to suprapubic catheterisation.

Once the bladder has been catheterised, allow it to drain freely. There is no need to clip and release the catheter in an attempt to prevent the bleeding which occurs rarely in patients with chronically obstructed systems.

Special Circumstances in Acute Retention

Constipation. Elderly frail men with mild prostatic obstruction may go into urinary retention if they become constipated. Unless they are in acute distress (and this is unusual) they should be initially treated by restoration of bowel function (for which a manual evacuation may be needed) and by mobilisation. Only if this fails should a catheter be passed.

Postoperative retention. There are three situations in the male:

1. Normal urethra but a painful perineal or lower abdominal procedure. Do not allow the bladder to become distended; if the patient cannot void after 16 hours pass a catheter, empty the bladder, relieve the pain and withdraw the catheter. Re-catheterisation is seldom necessary.

2. Same as above but mild or moderate prostatic obstruction. The catheter should be inserted as for the normal patient. However, it is best not to remove the catheter until the patient is able to stand, is reasonably active and has normal bowel function. If, even then, retention recurs then significant obstruction exists for which operation is required.

3. Damage to some component of the voiding mechanism, usually the motor nerves as a consequence of extensive pelvic dissection (e.g. abdominoperineal excision of the rectum). Here retention should nearly always be anticipated and bladder drainage instituted. Recovery is slow and continued catheterisation may be required for 7–10 days.

Stricture. The situation may be apparent from the history (e.g. past trauma; sexually transmitted disease; the slow onset of difficulty in voiding in a young man) or may be diagnosed at catheterisation by failure of the catheter to progress as far as the prostate. At all costs avoid further damage. Unless you have been trained, do not yourself undertake dilatation. Decompress suprapubically and seek help.

Postoperative Retention in Females

Postoperative retention is much less common in the female. However, there are a number of elderly women with chronically distended bladders, the cause of which is often uncertain. They may develop retention after operation. In these women it may be necessary to undertake a wide internal urethrotomy if they cannot void spontaneously after 2–3 days catheterisation.

Subsequent Management of Retention

Benign prostatic hypertrophy. In nearly all instances some form of prostatectomy should be undertaken as soon as possible. There is no need for 'emergency' prostatectomy; schedule the patient for the earliest operation list and thus avoid the complications of being in hospital, bed rest and prolonged catheterisation which include respiratory infections, venous thromboembolism and urinary tract infection.

The obstruction caused by the prostate can be overcome by either a transurethral or an open operation. There has been a very marked swing towards transurethral surgery. Open operations tend now to be performed only if the gland is very large or if there are multiple bladder stones in association with diverticula. Transurethral resection of the prostate is usually carried out under spinal or epidural anaesthesia. This has the advantage of causing minimal respiratory problems and it is often possible to detect complications at an earlier stage than would be the case if a general anaesthetic had been used.

Investigation and Preparation for Operation

The following investigations are the minimum which should be undertaken:

1. To assess renal function—serum creatinine, urea and electrolyte concentrations.

2. Urine culture at the time of catheterisation to ensure that there is no infection.

3. Haemoglobin or haematocrit to ensure that the patient is not anaemic, particularly if there is a significant degree of uraemia.

4. Blood group and match 2 units, though in some centres where blood is readily available grouping alone may be acceptable (see p. 68).

5. Chest x-ray.

6. Intravenous urogram. The value of this investigation is

debatable. It is unlikely to alter the need for or type of operation in benign prostatic hypertrophy and its main benefit will be to detect coexistent abnormalities. If there is a history of haematuria, recurrent infections or suspicion of a carcinoma of the prostate, then IV urography should be performed as it may help in diagnosis or staging.

7. Serum acid phosphatase concentration should be estimated if a carcinoma may be present. The enzyme is not of *diagnostic* value. Its major role is as a tumour marker to stage and monitor the progress of treatment of carcinoma of the prostate.

8. Prostatic biopsy. If the prostate feels malignant either aspiration or needle biopsy should be undertaken. Either a transperineal or transrectal approach can be used but if large needles are employed transrectally, an antibiotic which is effective against gram-negative organisms should be given for 12 hours.

9. Electrocardiogram in patients aged over 40.

10. The other important aspect of preparation is to explain to the patient the nature of the operation, by which route it will be performed and also that, after the operation, there will be significant amounts of blood in the urine for up to 2 weeks. It is also essential to allay fears regarding potency following prostatectomy, and to explain that retrograde ejaculation is an almost invariable sequel.

CARCINOMA OF THE PROSTATE

Management

The preoperative investigations are as for benign hypertrophy with the addition of a bone scintiscan.

Even if the diagnosis of carcinoma of the prostate is made preoperatively it is probably better to resect a passage than to treat with oestrogens for 10–14 days in the hope that this will cause sufficient shrinkage of the gland to overcome obstruction. A reasonable plan is to undertake, where medically possible, transurethral resection of the prostate in all men who present with retention caused by a carcinoma. If the serum acid phosphatase is normal and a bone scan negative, surgery is usually followed after 6 weeks by radiotherapy to the prostatic fossa and draining lymph nodes. The reason for waiting 6 weeks is to allow the prostatic fossa time to heal, as earlier irradiation will often lead to distressing frequency and urgency. It is also necessary to exclude infection before starting radiotherapy.

If the acid phosphatase is elevated or the bone scan is positive, or there is evidence detected by other means of spread beyond the prostate, radiotherapy should be abandoned in favour either of oestrogens, which should be given in a dose of stilboestrol 1 mg 3 times a day, or orchidectomy which will have substantially the same effect.

More recently, satisfactory androgen suppression has been achieved with LHRH antagonists. The advantage of this approach is that these drugs do not have oestrogenic side-effects and obviously avoid the psychological effects of surgical castration. Their major disadvantages are their high cost and inability to be taken orally.

There seems to be no place for a larger dose of oestrogens as maintenance therapy for this condition. A departure from this regimen should be considered only in the presence of severe ureteric obstruction with uraemia. In these circumstances it has been thought that high doses of oestrogen in the form of the synthetic agent fosfestrol (Honvan), 1 g/day for a week, may produce rapid shrinkage of the tumour and restoration of renal function. Unfortunately this treatment carries a high risk of venous thrombosis and heparin prophylaxis should be instituted (p.144) at the same time as oestrogen therapy. Suppression of testicular androgens has been the mainstay of treatment. However, recent studies have suggested that attempts should also be made to suppress adrenal androgens.

It is also possible that chemotherapy may supplement hormonal therapy but, at present, response rates with chemotherapy have been disappointing.

Management after Transurethral and Open Prostatectomy

The bladder is kept free of blood by means of catheter drainage, using a 24 or 26F Foley catheter. Some surgeons prefer to use a continuous irrigation system, relying on the free flow to prevent clotting. An irrigating system, however, is of little use once clots have occurred. Irrigating systems are best avoided if clot retention has occurred. An alternative method for managing patients postoperatively is to use a fluid load, together with diuretics, to ensure a good urine output. This has the disadvantage that, if not carefully managed, it may result in disturbances in fluid and electrolyte balance, particularly in elderly patients.

Management of Complications after Prostatectomy

Hypotension. This is probably the most common problem confronting a house surgeon dealing with patients who have had a prostatectomy. The major causes are blood loss and clot retention, bacteraemia and (much less commonly) myocardial infarction. The first step is personally to check the recordings of temperature, blood pressure and pulse rate, and to assess whether there is peripheral vasoconstriction. Then examine the catheter to see if it is draining adequately and to ascertain the nature of the fluid coming out and examine the abdomen to see if the bladder is distended.

Blood loss. That blood loss is the cause of hypotension is usually easily established. There will be a history of heavily blood-stained urine postoperatively with difficulty in maintaining drainage, and both will be apparent when the catheter bag is examined. There will often be clot retention (see below). In these circumstances it is necessary to replace blood, to ensure that there is free drainage from the bladder and to remove clots by bladder washout. If the closed drainage system has to be broken several times to wash out the bladder, antibiotics (directed against gram-negative organisms) should be given systemically.

Clot retention. In spite of the measures outlined above, bleeding can still be sufficiently severe to cause clots to form and result in retention. Do not be misled by clear through-and-through drainage, because often the clot prevents the irrigating fluid from reaching the bladder.

The clots can usually be cleared by a vigorous bladder washout using either normal saline or citrate solution. Using a Toomey or similar syringe, 50 ml of fluid should be instilled rapidly into the bladder. This will cause turbulence in the bladder and help to break up clots. The plunger of the syringe should be worked to and fro as this will help to propel the clots along the catheter. This process should be repeated until the clots have been removed and there is free drainage. If this technique is not successful, many simple manoeuvres such as letting down the balloon of the Foley catheter, or pushing the catheter further into the bladder, may be tried to improve drainage.

In general, it is preferable not to remove the catheter unless an experienced person is available or has advised this because it may be very difficult to re-insert, particularly after transurethral resection of the prostate. If the catheter is replaced then a size 24 or 26F should be used. It is important to stress that a full bladder is extremely painful and it is necessary to ensure that patients are given adequate pain relief if the obstruction cannot be cleared rapidly (p.25). Because of persistent severe bleeding, a small proportion of patients will need to return to theatre so that the bladder can be washed out using a large cystoscope or a resectoscope sheath. Sometimes bleeding in the immediate postoperative period can be controlled by over-inflating the Foley balloon with 40–50 ml of water and placing the catheter under traction—in some centres this is routine.

Bacteraemia. It is important always to be on the alert for this complication. The urinary tract is without doubt the most common source of bacteraemia. Patients should *not* undergo endoscopic or any other surgery on the prostate in the presence of an untreated infection.

The patient's temperature will be raised, he will have a tachycardia and possibly rigors; there will be a fall in blood pressure and peripheral cyanosis. When called to see such a patient it is important to assess his general condition. Ensure that he has an adequate fluid input. Elevate the foot of the bed and give oxygen via a face mask. Take blood for culture and give the 'best guess' antibiotic parenterally. Check that a urinary tract infection has not been overlooked before surgery. Organisms present in a preoperative culture will point to the correct diagnosis and also help in the selection of antibiotics to treat this condition.

For patients in severe shock it may be necessary to insert a central venous pressure catheter and to transfer them to an intensive therapy unit so that more intensive monitoring of cardiorespiratory function can be done. The condition requires rapid, aggressive treatment as it is potentially lethal (see p.148).

Special Complications of Transurethral Resection

Blood loss is more easily underestimated in endoscopic than in open prostatectomy because of the large volumes of irrigating fluid involved. Care must be taken to examine the irrigating fluid during operation and, because one is often dealing with frail, elderly men, blood replacement should be instituted before there are gross changes in pulse rate and blood pressure.

Fluid overload. Because of the nature of irrigating systems used during transurethral resection, large amounts of the irrigating fluid can be forced into the prostatic vessels and thus the systemic circulation. This can be minimised, but not totally prevented, by keeping the fluid reservoir no more than 60 cm above the operating table. Most units now use a 1.5% glycine solution which is isotonic. However, in some centres water is still used. In the case of glycine solution, a dilutional hyponatraemia occurs and if water is used this is aggravated by red cell lysis. Often the first indication that excessive fluid absorption is occurring is that the conscious patient under regional anaesthesia becomes agitated, restless and confused. The operation should be stopped, blood sent for serum sodium concentration and osmolality estimations, and 2% saline given intravenously. A large dose of a diuretic such as frusemide should be given intravenously as this will produce a diuresis with excretion of water in excess of electrolytes. Careful control of electrolyte balance is essential.

Bladder rupture or capsular perforation. Both conditions are usually detected during operation. The usual features are that the patient begins to complain of pain and the irrigating fluid does not seem to be returning properly. In these circumstances it may be necessary to make a suprapubic incision to drain the extravasated fluid and if necessary, repair the damage to the bladder.

RENAL CALCULI AND RENAL COLIC

Stones in the urinary tract are a common cause of acute surgical admission. Usually the patient has a stone arrested somewhere between the pelviureteric junction and the bladder.

The diagnosis of a ureteric calculus as a cause of severe abdominal pain is usually clear from the history, although at times this disorder may be confused with biliary colic, intestinal obstruction, appendicitis, leaking aortic aneurysm, hysteria, or a twisted ovarian cyst. There is a small group of patients who simulate renal colic in order to obtain narcotics (p.228). It is important to confirm the diagnosis as soon as possible, both in order positively to exclude other dangerous lesions and also to establish the effects the stone is producing on the kidney. If investigation is delayed the stone may pass so that when x-rays are taken nothing is found and the diagnosis remains in doubt.

Investigations

Microscopic examination of the urine. This should be performed on the first specimen of urine obtained. Almost invariably there will be red cells in the urine in the presence of renal colic. Although red cells may not be present, their absence casts doubt on the diagnosis.

Urine culture. It is important to exclude concurrent infection as the combination of complete or partial obstruction and infection can have rapid and disastrous effects on the kidneys.

Haematological and biochemical studies, particularly serum creatinine and calcium concentrations, should be obtained on admission.

An intravenous urogram (IVU) should be performed as soon as possible, preferably as the patient is passing through the A and E department. It is proper to do this, especially if there is diagnostic doubt, in spite of inadequate bowel preparation because the question 'Is there obstruction?' can usually be answered. Films taken at 5, 10 and 30 minutes will suffice and compression of the abdomen is not necessary. Thus the examination can be performed with the emergency room x-ray facilities. The IVU allows one to establish the diagnosis, to determine the size of the stone and also to tell the patient the likely course of management. In general, the size of the stone determines the management of the patient, assuming one is not dealing with specialised cases such as a solitary kidney or a stone in the presence of infection. Always make the point on the request form that the purpose of the investigation is to confirm a doubtful diagnosis. The three important signs on the affected side are:

1. Delayed excretion.

2. A 'nephrographic' effect—contrast medium outlining the renal substance.

3. An 'open' ureter down the side of obstruction, rather than the usual spindle.

Management of Renal Colic

Conservative

1. Pain relief. Pethidine provides adequate pain relief, but it is important to make sure that enough is given. Too often, small incremental doses are used which do not adequately overcome the pain. In fit young men 100 mg IM or an initial 50 mg IV should be the minimum dose.

2. Ensure that there is adequate fluid intake. This may not always be easy as there is frequently a degree of ileus associated with renal colic; it may then be necessary to give fluids intravenously.

3. Physical activity. Where possible the patient should be encouraged to remain ambulant.

Operative. In most instances the stone will pass spontaneously and as a working guide one can assume that 95% of stones of less than 5 mm in diameter will pass spontaneously, whereas only about 5% of stones greater than 10 mm in diameter will do so.

The other major indications for operative removal of a stone apart from size are:

1. A coexistent urinary tract infection.

2. A solitary kidney with impaired renal function.

3. Persistent severe pain with no radiological evidence of movement of the stone.

4. No symptoms, but where the stone has failed to progress over a period of no more than 6–8 weeks.

All patients who are to undergo surgery for stones should have a plain x-ray film of the whole urinary tract on the way to operation.

Until the last 5 years, apart from lower ureteric stones, the only satisfactory method for removal of a stone was an open operation. However, percutaneous techniques using an ultrasonic probe or shock waves generated outside the body which can be focused on the stone, can shatter a stone into tiny particles which can then pass spontaneously. This has meant that the need for open surgery has virtually disappeared in some centres. If these facilities are available the houseman will be required to arrange referral.

Late Management

Intravenous urogram. If a patient is being treated non-operatively it may be necessary to repeat the intravenous urogram, but in most cases a plain x-ray film is sufficient to show the progress or otherwise of opaque stones. If an operation has been performed it is important to ensure that there is free drainage and that the ureter has healed adequately. Ultrasound imaging may prove satisfactory for follow-up because in most cases one is looking for resolution of the pelvicaliceal dilatation caused by obstruction.

Urinary tract infection. Infection has to be excluded, but this largely applies to the follow-up of patients who have had staghorn calculi removed. In most other circumstances, unless there is some clinical indication, there should be no need to undertake routine urine cultures.

Biochemical investigation. The important objective is to find out if the patient has hyperparathyroidism. There are many ways of going about this but repeated serum calcium concentrations are the first line of investigation. At least three should be done over 2–3 weeks.

Treatment. After the first stone episode the patient should be advised to try to maintain a urine output of 1–1.5 litres per 24 hours. It is important to stress to the patient that his fluid intake is relatively irrelevant and that the important factor is the urine output. Patients should also be advised regarding diet, particularly those who have had calcium/oxalate stones. It is valuable to have available a diet sheet which lists the foods which are rich in calcium and oxalate.

Recurrent stones. The management of patients with recurrent stones may be helped by more extensive metabolic studies under controlled conditions and, depending on the findings, stone recurrences may be prevented by treatment with such agents as thiazides, cellulose phosphate or allopurinol.

MAJOR SURGERY ON THE URINARY TRACT

Apart from prostatectomy, already considered, and major operations on the kidney, the management of which corresponds to other abdominal procedures, the other major surgical assault is total cystectomy for bladder cancer. This operation may be difficult and bloody and, because of the ileal conduit, involves a change in life style. The following apply:

1. Make the patient aware of the problems of the ileal conduit and if there is a stoma service, enlist its help (p.210).

2. Ensure that the most appropriate site for the stoma is marked and that the mark will not be washed off by the agent used to prepare the skin prior to operation.

3. Warn the male patient of the inevitability of impotence.

4. Arrange for bowel preparation (p.209).

5. Order 6 units of blood (see p.68).

Chapter 23

Intestinal Obstruction

SMALL BOWEL OBSTRUCTION

Opinions differ as to whether a trial of conservative treatment with intravenous fluid replacement and gastric aspiration should always be undertaken. We believe that once the diagnosis is established, operative relief of the obstruction should be done as soon as the patient's condition permits. It is usually not possible to distinguish definitely on clinical grounds between a simple mechanical obstruction and bowel strangulation. However, in a patient with vague abdominal pain and perhaps only a few small bowel fluid levels on erect abdominal x-ray, the use of Gastrografin may allow a conservative policy to be pursued (see below). In the presence of strangulation, delay contributes to an immediately higher mortality.

History

1. Duration, site and character of the pain.
2. The character of the vomiting—whether it be of small quantity and therefore reflex in type, or of large volume suggesting mechanical regurgitation. Remember, vomiting will occur early in *upper* small bowel obstruction and will be delayed in distal obstruction.
3. When the patient's bowels moved last and when he last passed flatus.
4. The precise nature of any previous abdominal operations or symptoms suggestive of a progressive bowel lesion.
5. Enquire about the presence of a hernia and if it has become recently painful or irreducible.
6. Enquire regarding the ingestion of ganglion blocking or anti-depressant drugs.

Examination

Abdomen

1. Abdominal distension (often absent in early, high small bowel

obstruction, or closed loop obstruction).

2. Presence or absence of visible peristalsis.

3. Presence or absence of tenderness and guarding—may suggest strangulation.

4. Presence or absence of a succussion splash.

5. The character of bowel sounds and their relation to bouts of pain.

6. Presence or absence of hernia (inguinal, femoral, umbilical or incisional) and tenderness associated with it.

Rectal and/or vaginal examination

1. Determine presence of pelvic mass.

2. Determine whether rectum is full or empty.

Assessment of the patient's general condition to determine the amount of fluid replacement. This is dealt with more fully under fluid and electrolyte replacement (p. 87).

Investigations

1. *Abdominal x-rays.* Take x-rays before consideration of a sigmoidoscopy as insufflated air may confuse the picture. Erect and supine films should be taken though radiologists are less and less keen on the erect film. In general, the erect film is for the purpose of demonstrating fluid levels (remember that in children the presence of two or three small bowel fluid levels may be normal) and the supine film to determine the site of obstruction by means of bowel gas shadows. Order a PA chest x-ray at the same time.

In patients with vague abdominal pain and perhaps one or two fluid levels in whom the diagnosis of obstruction is not obvious (especially in those who have recurrent bouts of pain thought to be caused by intestinal adhesions) a Gastrografin study may be of value. Gastrografin (50 ml) is given by mouth and plain abdominal x-rays taken after 5 and 60 minutes. Passage of Gastrografin into the colon at 60 minutes indicates that if a degree of obstruction is present, it is only partial and conservative measures may be appropriate. Diarrhoea from the hypertonic agent may contribute to the relief of the obstruction.

2. Full blood count and creatinine and electrolytes. However, as pointed out under the heading of fluid and electrolyte replacement

(p. 83), with an obstruction of short duration these values may be normal and give no guide as to the extent of the fluid and electrolyte loss which may have occurred.

Preoperative Management

1. Analgesics.
2. A nasogastric tube may be inserted, and aspirated until the stomach is empty and placed on continuous drainage. However, do not rely on the nasogastric tube to have effectively emptied the stomach. Be on hand at the time of induction of anaesthesia to carry out cricoid compression so as to avoid reflux and inhalation (see p. 21).
3. An intravenous infusion is set up. In acute fluid loss there is no danger in rapid replacement, so at least half the estimated loss may be replaced rapidly in the first 1 or 2 hours before operation.
4. Prophylactic antibiotics are indicated. The suggested regimen is: metronidazole 500 mg IV, and cephazolin 500 mg IV with the premedication and two further doses intravenously 6 hours apart during the early postoperative period.

Postoperative Management

This is almost entirely a question of fluid and electrolyte replacement and maintenance. Early consideration should be given to nutrition and, if a prolonged period of recovery is anticipated, a subclavian feeding line is inserted early. Nasogastric or gastrostomy drainage is continued until bowel sounds are present, the patient has passed flatus and the volume of drainage is less than 300 ml/24 hours. When there is doubt if intestinal propulsion has returned to normal, 50 ml of water soluble contrast medium (e.g. Gastrografin) can be given either by mouth or tube. A film exposed at 1 hour should show the material in the distal small bowel and at 90 minutes in the caecum. Intake is then rapidly built up through clear fluids to mixed fluids and then to food.

LARGE BOWEL OBSTRUCTION

With the exception of sigmoid volvulus, large bowel obstruction and its features tend to develop more slowly than is the case with small bowel obstruction. The obstruction is essentially an acute-on-chronic type. Except where there is danger of rupture of the caecum there is, therefore, not the urgency with regard to operative treatment. Very occasionally conservative treatment is attempted, for if the bowel can be cleared and full bowel preparation carried out, planned surgery with a one-stage instead of a three-stage operation is feasible (see p. 209). However, there is currently a move to more aggressive resectional surgery as an emergency or semi-emergency for the chief cause of large bowel obstruction—cancer.

History

1. It is important to differentiate

    (a) acute volvulus with sudden onset of severe abdominal pain, and often gross distension

    (b) acute diverticulitis causing obstruction with a past history of similar attacks of pain in the left iliac fossa, and possibly diarrhoea

    (c) carcinoma, which is the commonest cause of obstruction with its attendant premonitory symptoms of change in bowel habit, weight loss, etc.

2. It is important to determine when the patient's bowels moved last and also when he last passed flatus.

Examination

Abdomen

1. Abdominal distension of a large bowel (peripheral) type.

2. Evidence of localised abdominal distension, i.e. is there a coil of sigmoid colon visible, suggesting a volvulus, or is the caecum visible, palpable or percussible?

3. The presence or absence of an abdominal mass.

4. The presence or absence of tenderness and guarding—suggesting, according to site, diverticulitis, sigmoid volvulus or danger of caecal rupture.

Rectal or vaginal examination. It is most important to attempt to detect the obstructing mass.

Assessment of patient's general condition. Vomiting is generally not prominent and while the patient may be ill, it is unusual for this to be the result of gross fluid and electrolyte loss.

Investigations

1. Abdominal x-rays—erect and supine. The supine film is important in determining the site of the obstruction from the gas shadows. PA chest x-ray.

2. Sigmoidoscopy—this should only be performed after x-rays have been taken as gas insufflation may confuse the picture. In subacute cases colonoscopy may be considered.

3. If the diagnosis of actual large bowel obstruction is in any way in doubt (and this is usual) an urgent Gastrografin enema should be performed. This may exclude patients with colonic 'pseudo-obstruction'—a dilated dysfunctioning colon, the result of multiple causes (e.g. recent hip surgery, severe respiratory infections).

4. Full blood count, creatinine and electrolytes, liver function tests. These are perhaps more important in the case of large bowel obstruction than small, because pre-existing anaemia or uraemia are not uncommon.

Treatment

1. In the case of a volvulus of the sigmoid colon, decompression of the bowel and reduction of the volvulus can usually be achieved by the passage of a flatus tube through a sigmoidoscope.

If these measures fail or are not applicable, laparotomy must be performed.

2. (a) For a carcinoma of the right side of the colon an emergency right hemicolectomy is generally performed, therefore blood (4 units) must be ready

(b) With the advent of on-table colonic irrigation it is becoming commoner for a left-sided carcinoma to be treated by an immediate resection with primary anastomosis (see p. 210). Alternatively, a Hartmann's resection is performed leaving a left iliac fossa colostomy with closure of the rectal stump.

In spite of these advances, the formation of a right transverse colostomy to decompress the bowel is still frequently the management used, permitting a planned resection some two weeks later.

(c) For volvulus, a Hartmann's resection is normally performed, i.e. radical sigmoid colectomy and closure of the rectal stump

(d) For an obstruction caused by diverticulitis, management is as for (b). Anastomoses may be marked with metal clips to allow visualisation or postoperative contrast studies.

Preoperative Management

In acute large bowel obstruction this is as for small bowel obstruction except that for antibiotic prophylaxis the following regimen is suggested: gentamicin 2 mg/kg and metronidazole 500 mg are given IV with the premedication with two further doses administered 6 hourly during the early postoperative period. Note: gentamicin is given in a dose of 1 mg/kg postoperatively (see p. 128).

Postoperative Management

This generally presents less of a problem than with small bowel obstruction. Intravenous fluid therapy may be expected to continue for only 24–48 hours. When a colostomy is present, oral fluids may be commenced when this has worked.

Consider performing a contrast Gastrografin study on the eighth postoperative day to outline the anastomosis (this has usually been marked with metal clips—unnecessary if a stapled anastomosis has been performed). See 'Large Bowel Surgery' for details of contrast study.

Large Bowel Surgery

Most surgery is carried out for cancer and inflammatory disease. Apart from the general preoperative measures common to all major surgery the most important consideration is that the large bowel should be empty at the time of surgery. Not only does this make the procedure safer but also it makes it possible to avoid a temporary colostomy or ileostomy proximal to a suture line.

PREOPERATIVE INVESTIGATIONS

General:

1. Full blood count, creatinine and electrolytes, liver function tests.

2. Baseline blood gases and respiratory function tests.

3. Chest x-ray and ECG.

4. Double contrast barium enema—this will have been performed in the outpatient clinic. Check that the films are available.

5. Sigmoidoscopy and/or colonoscopy—this will have been undertaken in the outpatient clinic and biopsies taken. Check that you have a report on all biopsies taken.

6. Preoperative IVU has recently been shown to be of little value in detecting ureteric involvement by tumour and thus its use is no longer recommended.

BOWEL PREPARATION

Surgeons are very individualistic about this as with many other things.

1. In the unobstructed case either antegrade or retrograde techniques may be used. Most surgeons prefer the former with either:

(a) *Whole gut irrigation.* A nasogastric tube is passed and the patient sits on a commode. Diazepam 5 mg and metoclopramide 10 mg IM may be given. A measured 3 litres of normal saline are given hourly down the tube until the rectal effluent is clear (usually 8–10 litres). This may be a tiring procedure in the elderly though there is not much risk of heart failure.

(b) *Cathartics*. A wide variety is used. Currently bisocodyl or sodium picosulphate (Picolax in the UK) are most popular given on the day before operation. The danger here is dehydration and the patient should drink copiously or have intravenous supplements if signs of extracellular deficiency are noted.

Techniques of using cathartics vary. One example:

On operation day minus 2: patient is admitted to hospital, eats a normal ward diet and that evening is given 2 bisacodyl tablets.

On operation day minus 1: has a normal breakfast but thereafter has a liquid diet. At 10:00 h, 350 ml of magnesium citrate solution (USNF) are sipped over an hour or so. That evening a phosphate enema is given.

Operation day: nil by mouth and at 06:00 h the patient is given a high colonic lavage until the return is clear.

Picolax has found much favour both for colonoscopy preparation and before surgery.

Colonoscopy

Low fibre diet for 48 hours pre examination.
Picolax one sachet at 20:00 h day prior to examination then clear fluids only.
Picolax one sachet at 08:00 h on day of examination then water only.

Major Large Bowel Surgery

Fluids only for 24 hours.
Picolax one sachet at 08:00 h on day prior to operation.
Picolax one sachet at 14:00 h on day prior to operation, then clear fluids only.

Rectal and Anal Surgery

Picolax one sachet at 20:00 h the night before operation.
Phosphate enema 3 hours pre-op.

Retrograde irrigation—'high enemas', 'colonic lavage'—is less commonly used. The techniques are always those of the individual team or unit and so will not be detailed here. An obstructed patient (and note that this does not mean exclusively those with acute obstruction) may be prepared by 'on table irrigation'. The technique has two advantages: first, during emergency surgery for the obstructed large bowel it allows rapid clearance of the faecal load permitting primary anastomosis and lowering the defunctioning colostomy rate. Second, it enables clear bowel to be examined endoscopically at operation. Some surgeons have come to use the techniques almost routinely and this avoids the rigours of preoperative preparation for the patient. The houseman should warn the operating room staff that it may be needed. Firstly if a decompressing colostomy has already been done, the patient's distal colon is washed out from the anus and through the colostomy until the return from both ends is clear; water may be used for this purpose. At the same time one of the regimens outlined above is used on the proximal bowel to reduce the problems of perioperative soiling of the operation field. Low colorectal anastomosis is now being performed more frequently and the anal sphincter is preserved thus reducing the need for colostomies.

Stoma care has improved greatly over the last few years. Not only have appliances and adhesives improved, but also nurses who specialise in the care of these patients—stoma therapists—are increasing in number. When such a person is available she should be consulted several days *before* operation. She will share with the medical staff the burden of explanation to the patient (but remember it is difficult for anyone to comprehend a stoma until he or she has one) and may also bring along a successful stoma patient to talk to your patient and instil confidence. The therapist will select the site most suitable for the opening. An adhesive face plate will then be attached to this site and the patient should wear it for a night and a day so that adjustments can be made if the site is found not to be optimal. Stoma therapists should work in concert with the surgical team and their presence is not an excuse to subcontract every detail of management to them.

Prophylactic Antibiotics

Gentamicin 2 mg/kg and metronidazole 500 mg are given IV with the premedication and again as two further doses 6 hours apart in the postoperative period. The postoperative dose of gentamicin is 1 mg/kg.

PLANNED PROCEDURES: COLON

Right hemicolectomy. This is performed for a lesion of the terminal ileum or right side of the colon as far as the hepatic flexure. For a lesion of the transverse colon or hepatic flexure an *extended right hemicolectomy* may be performed. Even in the presence of obstruction, this is carried out as a one-stage procedure.

Transverse colectomy. This is an uncommon operation now—extended right hemicolectomy is preferred.

Left hemicolectomy and sigmoid colectomy. Performed for curative resection of left-sided colonic lesions. It may be performed as a primary procedure or following a defunctioning right transverse colostomy.

PLANNED PROCEDURES: RECTUM

There are two standard procedures in use.

Anterior restorative resection. This is a resection and end-to-end anastomosis with preservation of the lower rectum and sphincter, performed by the abdominal route. It is the procedure of choice for sigmoid diverticulitar disease and is used in selected cases of carcinoma. In the past this operation has not been performed if the growth is less than 8 cm from the anus. However, with the circular stapling devices now available lower resections are possible. The two chief dangers are:

1. Anastomotic leak—this may be clinically apparent, with the development of faecal peritonitis or a pelvic abscess, or only detected radiologically after contrast examination of the

anastomosis.

2. Obstruction at the anastomosis. A careful watch must be kept for abdominal distension for the first few days. A supine abdominal x-ray may be useful to distinguish small bowel distension (ileus) from large bowel (obstruction).

Abdomino-perineal excision of rectum. Used when anterior resection is not possible. The simultaneous combined operation is undertaken, except where hip movement is so limited that adequate simultaneous exposure is impossible.

POSTOPERATIVE MANAGEMENT

With the exception of operations on the left side, where catheterisation is routine and special attention to the perineal wound is required, the postoperative management is much the same as for small bowel surgery. Techniques for managing perineal wounds are very individual.

Contrast Studies of the Anastomosis

These may be performed on the eighth postoperative day to test for anastomotic leakage. Gastrografin is the contrast medium of choice and may be administered in two ways:

1. Retrograde—a Gastrografin enema performed using a *soft* rubber catheter and careful technique.

2. Antegrade—if on-table colonic irrigation has been performed prior to anastomosis, the Foley catheter inserted into the caecum or terminal ileum is left in place. Gastrografin may then be instilled into the colon via this catheter to image the anastomosis.

It is essential that you accompany the patient to the x-ray department to explain the surgical anatomy to the radiologist and ensure *gentle* technique.

Chapter 25

Acute Pancreatitis

The diagnosis of acute pancreatitis would appear to be quite straightforward but this is often not the case. If a patient with acute abdominal pain has a serum amylase greater than 1000 IU/l, pancreatitis is the most likely diagnosis. However, hyper-amylasaemia per se does not mean that the patient has histological change in the pancreas amounting to acute pancreatitis.

The picture becomes complicated as:

1. 5% of patients with acute pancreatitis have a serum amylase within the normal range

2. Other conditions which cause acute abdominal pain can also cause hyperamylasaemia (usually, but not invariably, less than 1000 IU/l).

These conditions include:

    (a) perforated peptic ulcer
    (b) acute cholecystitis
    (c) mesenteric infarction
    (d) leaking abdominal aortic aneurysm.

Thus the differential diagnosis needs to be considered and the label of acute pancreatitis applied only after exclusion of these causes.

History

It is important to enquire about:

1. The nature, onset and radiation of the pain—pain radiating through to the back may be caused by pancreatitis *or* a posteriorly penetrating peptic ulcer; pain referred to the shoulder tip is indicative of a perforated peptic ulcer.

2. A history of previous attacks of similar pain and precipitating factors (e.g. alcoholic binge). Also results of relevant investigations performed previously.

3. A history of peptic ulceration or gall stones.

4. Drug history—frusemide, corticosteroids, azathioprine and amphetamines are all thought to cause pancreatitis.

5. Alcohol intake.

Examination

1. General examination—look for jaundice and signs of alcoholic liver disease.

2. Assess circulatory state and the degree of dehydration.

3. Abdomen—generalised tenderness and guarding are the usual findings, although this may be limited to the upper abdomen. Tenderness over the left loin on percussion (over the tail of the pancreas) can often be elicited. Grey Turner's sign and Cullen's sign, both the outcome of staining by tissue necrosis along extraperitoneal planes, are rare and only occur late in haemorrhagic pancreatitis.

Management

This can be divided thus:

1. Initial investigation
   (a) assessment of severity
   (b) cause
2. Fluid management and analgesia.

Initial Investigations

1. Full blood count, haematocrit, creatinine and electrolytes and liver function tests

2. Serum amylase, calcium and blood glucose

3. Blood gases (baseline)—a low Pa_{O_2} is not an uncommon finding in early acute pancreatitis

4. Erect PA chest x-ray—look for pneumoperitoneum. This also serves as a baseline for comparison of subsequent chest x-rays.

Assessment of severity. A severe attack which will require consideration of intensive care is defined in the first 48 hours by the presence of three or more of the following criteria:

1. White cell count $> 16 \times 10^9/l$
2. Blood glucose > 10 mmol/l
3. Serum calcium < 2.0 mmol/l
4. Rising blood urea (> 16 mmol/l). Creatinine gives the same information.
5. Reduced arterial oxygen tension ($Pa_{O_2} < 60$ mmHg = 8 kPa)
6. Base deficit > 4 mmol
7. Falling haematocrit (3% or more/48 hours)
8. Fluid requirement greater than 6 litres in 48 hours.

Aetiology. Although the determination of the aetiology of acute pancreatitis is important, it is only of necessity in immediate management to exclude the presence of gall stones as early surgery may be indicated in gall stone pancreatitis. Biliary excretion scan (HIDA) is the investigation of choice and if the gall bladder is not visualised at 60 minutes, gall stone pancreatitis is likely. Ultrasound of the gall bladder may be useful if HIDA scanning is not available, but its sensitivity is often limited by dilatation of the gas-filled transverse colon which obscures the biliary anatomy. Abdominal CT scan is rapidly becoming the most useful investigation in acute pancreatitis as it will not only indicate the presence of gall stones but will also give the degree of pancreatic involvement and used serially will give information on necrosis of the gland and the development of extrapancreatic collections (i.e. pseudocysts).

Fluid Management and Analgesia

Administer morphine by intravenous infusion (p. 25). Set up a reliable intravenous line and in severe cases a subclavian line for fluid infusion and CVP monitoring. Consider the insertion of a subclavian line for parenteral nutrition at the same time.

Administer Hartmann's solution to restore circulatory stability. The use of a nasogastric tube is controversial and is probably not necessary unless the patient is vomiting. Institute nil by mouth. Agents such as aprotinin (Trasylol) and glucagon have not been shown to be of any value.

Continued Management

Early operation may be undertaken in gall stone pancreatitis—have blood available and arrange for an operative cholangiogram. Monitor temperature, blood pressure and pulse and examine the abdomen at least twice a day. Consider TPN in prolonged ileus.

Repeat the following investigations daily:

1. Full blood count
2. Creatinine and electrolytes
3. Serum amylase (until normal)
4. Blood gases
5. Serum calcium
6. Blood glucose.

Check the following twice weekly:

1. Liver function tests
2. Chest x-ray.

Serial abdominal CT scans may be performed if available.

Progressive respiratory insufficiency (this may develop quite insidiously) will require ventilation. Deterioration in the above indices and continuing fever and tachycardia should be indications for your senior to decide on early operative intervention and excision of the necrotic pancreatic tissue.

Chapter 26

Thyroid and Parathyroid Surgery

THYROID

History

1. *Duration* of the goitre and *recent change in its size,* as well as *recent change in voice, difficulty with swallowing, cough, shortness of breath.*

2. Cardinal symptoms of *hyperthyroidism* should be enquired for.

3. What *drugs* have been taken? For how long?

4. The *locality* in which the patient was born and spent his/her early life should be recorded, together with the presence or absence of goitre among other members of the family.

Examination

1. The *size* of the goitre.

2. Its *consistency*, and whether it is *diffuse or nodular.*

3. Is there an *intrathoracic extension*? Make the patient cough.

4. Is there *tracheal compression,* as judged by wheezing on hyperextension or other movement of the neck?

5. Is there *venous obstruction*, i.e. distended veins of neck? Distinct congestion of head and neck caused by stretching hands above head? May also accentuate tracheal compression.

6. Is there *voice change* suggestive of recurrent laryngeal nerve involvement?

7. Is there a *Horner's syndrome* suggestive of cervical sympathetic involvement?

8. Is there clinical evidence of *hyperthyroidism*, e.g. exophthalmos, sleeping tachycardia, obvious weight loss, machinery bruit over thyroid suggesting multiple A-V fistulae, onycholisis, vitiligo.

Investigations

1. Haematology screen.

2. PA chest and *lordotic views of neck and thoracic inlet* for tracheal deviation and compression.

3. Laryngoscopy—indirect by arrangement with the ENT department:

    (a) a cord palsy *may* signify carcinoma

    (b) as a record to compare with postoperative appearance.

4. Ultrasound to delineate cysts.

5. Hyperthyroidism. In most patients the diagnosis will have been established but if investigations are required:

    (a) sleeping pulse rate

    (b) thyroid function tests. Never rely on a single test. Remember to elicit menstrual history, and history of iodine intake by mouth or exposure to iodine-containing contrast media, before ^{131}I uptake and ^{131}I scanning. Oestrogens or contraceptive pill affect T4 levels.

6. A serum calcium and phosphate concentration in any patient who is to undergo surgery.

7. Scanning. A thyroid gamma scan is not now generally regarded as vital, but from time to time gives useful information on two counts:

    (a) anatomy

    (b) the presence or absence of uptake in the nodule or nodules. If a 'cold' nodule is revealed by gamma scanning, a cyst may be distinguished from a solid tumour (? neoplasm) by ultrasound scanning.

8. Fine needle aspiration cytology. In many centres this has become the initial investigation of choice for a nodule in the thyroid. It can distinguish cyst from solid and frequently give a definite answer on whether benign or malignant disease is present. It has good specificity for papillary malignancy; 30% of atypical aspirates demonstrate malignancy in operative specimen.

Preoperative Preparation

In euthyroid patients no special preparation will be required. In hyperthyroid patients the preparation will generally have been carbimazole 10 mg every 8 hours, reduced when full control is reached. If control is difficult and the patient becomes hypothyroid, add thyroxine 0.1–0.15 mg to carbimazole. Preoperative preparation may also include 10 drops of Lugol's iodine (in milk) t.d.s. for 10–14 days to make the gland less vascular. This can be given together with carbimazole. Propranolol or other beta-blocking drugs may also be used. Some units rely on propranolol given in doses of up to 120 mg/day controlled by sleeping pulse which should fall to below 70/minute. When propranolol is used as preparation, it should be continued for 3–4 days after surgery, as its sudden cessation postoperatively may be associated with thyroid storm.

When a patient has a single nodule a frozen section should be arranged.

Postoperative Management

This is uncomplicated in most cases. There are certain complications, however, which require emergency treatment.

1. Haemorrhage into the pretracheal space with asphyxia. The emergency treatment consists of the immediate removal, in the patients's bed, of skin and deep sutures to permit separation of the strap muscles and evacuation of clot.

2. Bilateral recurrent laryngeal nerve damage is very rare but may produce sufficient restriction of airway to necessitate emergency tracheostomy.

3. Hypoparathyroidism. This may occasionally occur as a complication of any bilateral thyroidectomy but more particularly after total thyroidectomy for carcinoma and following pharyngolaryngectomy. It is important to perform a biochemical screen which includes serum calcium concentration before operation, and on the day after operation. A marked postoperative fall should lead to daily estimation of serum calcium concentration until serum calcium is normal or supportive medication is judged necessary. A watch should be kept, at least daily, for signs of impending tetany. Ask the patient if he/she has a feeling of tingling around the mouth. Tap the skin over the facial nerve gently with the finger tip; a twitch in the facial muscles suggests marked hypocalcaemia:

(a) in acute postoperative hypocalcaemia, intravenous calcium gluconate infusion (starting with 10 ml of 10% solution) is necessary and 1,25 dihydroxy vitamin D 0.25 mg twice daily will often assist in rapid stabilisation before introducing long-term therapy as outlined

(b) for long-term therapy, give 4–20 g calcium by mouth daily as effervescent tablets of calcium gluconate or calcium tartrate powder (not tablets as they are not absorbed). Calciferol 100 000 units daily or dihydrotachysterol (AT 10) 0.75–2.5

mg daily (3-10 ml or 6-20 capsules).

4. Thyroid storm or crisis. This should never occur if the patient is properly prepared. Recognised by agitation, delirium, hyperthermia, tachycardia and hypotension. The most important therapy is intravenous propranolol (0.5-1 mg) or similar agent and the surgery of hyperparathryoidism should not be undertaken (particularly if beta-blockers are used for preoperative preparation) without this agent being available. Supportive measures include cold sponging or ice bath, IV saline, oxygen, and chlorpromazine or diazepam in small doses IV. Summon help.

PARATHYROID

Surgery is undertaken only for hyperparathyroidism and is largely the task of highly specialised units. The general preparation is the same as for thyroid surgery with the addition of specialised suppression and imaging tests.

Chapter 27

Transthoracic Surgery

In a general surgical unit the most common conditions for which a thoracic approach is used are hiatus hernia, carcinoma or stricture of the lower end of the oesophagus, and carcinoma of the cardiac end of the stomach. In the first of these conditions a purely thoracic approach will be employed; in the others either an abdomino-thoracic or an abdominal followed by a separate thoracic exposure.

Preoperative Management

1. Great attention must be paid to *preoperative breathing exercises* so that the patient may establish a routine which is carried on after operation.
2. Stop the patient smoking.
3. Assess respiratory function by VC, FEV, and baseline arterial blood gases.
4. Treat any existing lung infection. Delay elective operation until the lung is clear. Patients with chronic lung disease may require an extended period of physiotherapy (e.g. 1 week).

Postoperative Management

Underwater drain. The purpose of this is to ensure that a negative intrapleural pressure exists and therefore full lung expansion will result, while permitting the drainage of blood or exudate. The fluid level in the drain will normally fluctuate with respiration; if it does not, either:

1. The lung has fully re-expanded.
2. The drain itself is blocked with blood clot.

It is a good routine practice to put a chest drain on low pressure suction (-4 or -5 mmHg) for at least the first 24 hours. Such a drain will not 'swing'.

Rules for removal of the chest drain vary from unit to unit.

General guidelines: full expansion demonstrated radiologically for 24 hours; output of serum less than 150 ml/24 hours; no concurrent need for drainage, e.g. an anastomosis. The lungs should be fully expanded within a few hours of operation and remain so. Therefore a *chest x-ray* must be taken and inspected on the *evening of the operation,* on the *two successive days* and at less frequent intervals until the patient is fully convalescent. If at any time there are clinical and radiological signs of *pulmonary collapse,* urgent measures must be taken. The first is the active *personal* encouragement of the patient to cough up retained sputum and energetic professional physiotherapy. If this produces improvement conservative measures are persisted with. If there is, however, no improvement, immediate *bronchoscopy* may be necessary and advice should be sought, particularly if there is audible bubbling in the airways.

CHEST INJURIES

Their importance lies not so much in the anatomical nature of the lesions, as in their effect on present and future respiratory function.

Examination

1. Rib fractures are detected by systematic palpation for local pain or crepitus.

2. It is most important to look for *paradoxical movement* of portions of the rib cage: *flail chest.*

3. Tension pneumothorax, or increasing pneumothorax, must be watched for. Tracheal deviation to the *unaffected* side is of particular significance.

4. Subcutaneous emphysema is almost always the result of puncture of the lung but may indicate rupture of a major airway, e.g. trachea or very occasionally of the oesophagus. Early bronchoscopy may be indicated.

5. A pericardial friction rub can indicate bruising of the heart.

6. The presence of, or an increasing degree of, haemothorax must be assessed and drainage instituted.

Investigations

1. Erect PA or AP x-rays are most important. There is rarely, if

ever, a contraindication to sitting the patient up momentarily to take an erect picture but the house surgeon will personally have to see that this is done in severely ill patients. Supine films can show considerable blood loss but they are usually misinterpreted because they show an even, gradual greying and whitening out of the lung field.

Watch particularly for the broadening of the mediastinum which may be the result of a tear of the aorta.

2. In all except the most trivial injuries baseline (and usually repeated) arterial blood gas studies should be done.

3. In complicated circumstances it is good practice to insert either a central venous line or a Swan Ganz catheter to measure central pressures.

Treatment

1. Intensive prophylactic physiotherapy to avoid sputum retention.

2. Adequate relief of pain. Continuous intravenous morphine at the appropriate carefully supervised dose does *not* cause respiratory depression. Unrelieved pain promotes shallow respiration, poor compliance to physiotherapy and sputum retention.

3. Prophylactic antibiotics should be given to anyone with a chest injury who has a previous history of chest infection or disease. They are *not* recommended in the healthy.

4. Multiple rib fractures, particularly if the result of a crushing injury, are frequently associated with heavy compression of the lungs, resulting in bruising and patchy consolidation, which takes some time to recover. It is the underlying lung injury which, as much as the mechanical damage to breathing, may call for ventilation. If the lung contusion is severe some surgeons use diuretics and steroids but this is controversial.

Do not forget that a patient with a chest injury and on a ventilator needs food and water.

5. Tension pneumothorax. This takes priority over everything else. The houseman may have to insert a wide bore needle in the third interspace anteriorly to save life. In less dramatic circumstances formal chest drainage is done urgently (p. 106).

6. Haemothorax: insertion of underwater pleural drain, and blood transfusion. Penetrating injuries may continue to bleed after

the insertion of a chest drain; thoracotomy is then required.

As a simple guide thoracotomy will probably be indicated if blood is lost in any of the following combinations: 500 ml of blood in 1 hour, 400 ml of blood for 2 consecutive hours, 300 ml of blood for 3 consecutive hours and 200 ml of blood for 4 consecutive hours or a total of 1 litre in 4 hours.

Chapter 28

Sexually Transmitted Disease

Since the mid-1950s there has been a significant increase in the incidence of venereal disease. Consequently, the possibility of venereal disease always must be considered in patients presenting with urethral symptoms. While it is true that most sexually transmitted infections involve the genitals, infection of the rectum, pharynx and conjunctiva are common. The most frequent source of venereal disease is a 'casual' sexual partner. However, if the dissemination of this disease through the community is to be minimised, every attempt should be made to treat every sexual partner of the patient.

Investigation

Most patients will present with a urethral discharge, a penile lesion or a vaginal discharge. In the case of the male, a smear of the discharge should be made and a Gram stain performed. If negative for gonococcus, then culture on a selective medium (available in most hospitals) should be undertaken. In females an endocervical swab should be taken and the swab rolled onto a culture medium that can be incubated in a CO_2-enriched atmosphere. If specific culture media are not available Stuart's transport medium can be used, but the recovery of gonococci will be reduced. However, Stuart's medium is satisfactory for culturing *Trichomonas* which causes similar symptoms to gonococcus in women. Failure to demonstrate or grow gonococci in the presence of a purulent urethral discharge is usually sufficient to make a diagnosis of non-specific urethritis. If further refinement in diagnosis is required then specific culture media are available for the isolation of *Chlamydia*.

When syphilis is suspected on the basis of the history and the examination, dark field microscopy is the preferred diagnostic test. If possible, the patient should be directed to the laboratory for collection of the specimen as examination should take place as soon as possible. Failure to see organisms necessitates serological investigation to provide indirect evidence to support the clinical diagnosis. The recommended tests are the non-treponemal, VDRL and the treponemal tests FTA-ABS (fluorescent treponemal antibody absorption test).

In the case of genital herpes, the presence of a small group of vesicles with bright red areolae, or discrete erosions which are painful and tender, should alert the clinician to the possibility of herpes. If required, plain swabs of material from the vesicles and erosions can be placed in viral transport medium for identification by an appropriate laboratory.

Treatment

Gonorrhoea: ampicillin 3.5 g orally and probenecid 1.0 g orally.
Syphilis: benzanthine penicillin G 1.8 g by IM injection.
Non-specific urethritis: tetracycline 500 mg orally 6 hourly for 7 days.
Trichomoniasis, chlamydia: metronidazole 2.0 g as a single oral dose.

All treatment to be discontinued at 48 hours.

ACQUIRED IMMUNE DEFICIENCY SYNDROME (AIDS)

The house surgeon may encounter this condition or its antecedent —antigen positivity to HI virus—in two ways: first because patients with AIDS develop complications which may require surgical treatment; second because he has to treat patients in high risk groups who have surgical problems. Chief among the latter are homosexuals with anorectal disorders.

Stringent rules govern the handling of patients who have AIDS though these may vary from place to place. In general the precautions observed are the same as those for patients who are carriers of hepatitis B virus. Special care should be taken to avoid splashing of secretions into the eyes: visors are usually recommended for operations or minor procedures.

Patients who are possibly HIV positive are in a more controversial group. On the one hand, it is useful for the surgical team to know that this is so because of the slightly increased risk (but it is very slight) that goes with looking after such people. On the other hand, for someone to discover that he or she is HIV positive can be a serious threat to his existence because upwards of 40% or more go on to develop AIDS. Do not undertake screening of patients for HIV positivity without consultation with your seniors.

There are counselling services available to patients with these sexually transmitted viral conditions and you should know how these can be contacted.

Chapter 29

Inner City Patients and Other Social Problems

Those who work in inner city hospitals in the 1980s are likely to come across distinct groups of patients who will present with real or simulated surgical emergencies. Other social problems arise in all communities.

MUNCHAUSEN SYNDROME

This term, originally coined by Richard Asher, describes a patient whose history is so dramatic that it is either compelling, impossible or both (e.g. the original patient had had his many abdominal operations in a Japanese prisoner of war camp and his abdomen closed with string from Red Cross parcels), and whose signs are real but often out of tune with his/her demeanour. Though obviously not addicts, they frequently welcome opiates; are shifty about personal background; demanding of attention; and likely to take their own discharge. The houseman's job is to be aware of this problem and if a previous hospital admission is quoted to follow that up urgently (see p.5). Their importance is that they must be distinguished from real *surgical* emergencies.

DRUG ADDICTS

The usual causes of surgical admission are:

1. Superficial or deep venous thrombosis, often with a septic element.
2. Subcutaneous sepsis.

Both require treatment on their merits. However, do not look for compliance or gratitude in these patients—they are interested in survival and where the next 'fix' is coming from. Referral to social workers and addiction centres is routine but rarely effective.
3. Remember that these patients have a high incidence of HIV and hepatitis B infection.

ROUGH SLEEPERS

All cities have a population of those who are 'of no fixed abode'.
They develop septic complications and hypothermia, both of which
require treatment. They are usually keen to get out and back to
their usual domicile. Social services have little to offer.

Chapter 30

Forensic Problems

House surgeons do not often encounter situations with legal overtones which are so acute that they are unable to get advice from their seniors, which should always be obtained. It is worth realising that a lack of expedition and of suspicion on the part of the house surgeon may embarrass future legal manoeuvres to help the patient or to see that justice is done. House surgeons must realise that in each situation the management of the patient must be placed before any broader societal considerations or responsibilities that may be thrust upon them by police or social workers who are interested in the case.

In all instances make written notes, preferably at the time rather than later. Written notes may be augmented by good quality, well-lit, black and white or colour photography. The names of witnesses should always be recorded in the patient's notes and any relevant timings should be recorded also.

SUSPICIOUS CIRCUMSTANCES

There are three:

Road traffic accidents, in which either the driver or a pedestrian is injured, may be associated with alcohol or drug abuse.

Child abuse is not an uncommon problem nowadays and unless the house surgeon is on the ball, the abused child may be allowed home to be further damaged, perhaps fatally.

Cases of physical assault and of *alleged sexual interference* also come into A and E departments.

ROAD TRAFFIC ACCIDENTS

At least 20 people are likely to die each day on the roads in the UK and many more will be injured. Similar figures apply almost anywhere in the Western World. Many of the injured will be removed by ambulance and brought to hospital where the first opportunity for them to be examined by a doctor will occur. Most are 'real' road traffic accidents but occasionally a road traffic accident may be staged as a deliberate attempt to conceal an assault, a homicide or a suicide.

In the UK the putative driver involved in a road traffic accident is subject to the drink and driving provisions of the Road Traffic Act, 1972, and similar rules are in force elsewhere. The police may require the driver to have his blood alcohol estimated. Obtaining the specimens for this is a police matter. However, the house surgeon must protect his patient's (and his own!) interests and should always try to obtain blood for alcohol estimation, particularly in an unconscious patient; a low blood alcohol may have a positive effect by protecting the patient from unwarranted prosecution. A blood alcohol level determined in an unconscious patient can only be used to assist in *medical management* unless the patient gives legal consent subsequently. Any pedestrian injured or killed in a road traffic accident should also have his blood analysed for alcohol as a protection for the motorist. Elsewhere in the world blood alcohol determinations are a legal requirement in all motorcar accidents.

Careful notes must be made of the time the casualty was brought to hospital and the time that the house surgeon first saw and examined the patient. The state of the patient on arrival, whether conscious, unconscious, disorientated or rational; did he have any other injuries and careful details of measurements of all injuries should be made and written down. Photographs should be taken of injuries, insofar as it is possible, but in particular, disfiguring facial injuries which are likely to be the subject of litigation at a later date should be photographed both before and after immediate surgical treatment.

CHILD ABUSE

Child abuse may consist of physical injury when injury was inflicted or not knowingly prevented by a person having custody or care of the child. This includes cases where poisonous or noxious substances have been administered to a child and physical neglect when the victim has been exposed to cold or starvation. Emotional or mental abuse is a further category and children so suffering may present as a 'failure to thrive'. It must be stressed that if one sibling in a house is suspected of suffering abuse, it is always advisable that the other children in the house should be examined.

The diagnosis is made by being suspicious and then carefully examining the child. Suspicions should always be aroused if injuries are incompatible with history or if the interval between the accident and reporting is prolonged. Good records must be kept of the time the child was examined, who brought the child to the doctor, what history was given by the parents and what history was given, if one was available, from the child. A full physical examination and urinalysis (especially for blood) must be made and photographs should be taken of any bruises. If the child is bruised and has injuries, x-rays of ribs, spine, limbs and head should always be taken to identify recent or old fractures which may indicate the time scale of the problem. It is useful to screen for clotting disorders.

If there is a reasonable doubt that the injuries are not purely accidental, the child should be admitted forthwith to a paediatric department. After this, a senior colleague must be consulted, the Register/Index of Non-Accidental Injuries interrogated and the designated nursing staff/social worker informed. All health authorities in the UK have published policies for the management of non-accidental injuries to children whereby the police and the social services department are involved and a case conference called. Usually by this stage the house surgeon will have nothing further to do other than to report the findings that were apparent when the child was brought to hospital. Similar rules apply elsewhere.

Where other children are involved in the household, it may be necessary to make immediate arrangements for them to be examined and protected. In such cases it is best to have the child kept occupied and supervised by the nurses in hospital while you go elsewhere and alert your senior colleagues, the designated nursing staff and the social services department about the problem. The social services department has the statutory obligation to place all the children in a protected environment.

ASSAULT

Any medical practitioner may find himself called upon to examine a person who has sustained an injury of some nature and he may, at a later date, be required to report upon the injury and its possible sequelae either in criminal proceedings or in pursuit of a civil claim for compensation. Violence is everywhere on the increase; cases of injury are now commonplace at football matches and similar sporting gatherings, including riots, and these may come under the management of a house surgeon at any time.

Other injuries that are important include firearm injuries and stab wounds. The important role of the house surgeon is in the correct recording of information, particularly when the patient first presents. Wounds are best divided into five categories: bruises, abrasions, lacerations, incisions and stab wounds, and each of these must be measured and described carefully. If possible the description should be aided by photographs. The colour of the bruises is important because this gives some indication of the time that they have been present. Scalds and burns are also wounds that may have been inflicted upon a person and careful details of their extent and their depth is vital. In the case of a minor, the written consent of a parent, guardian or close relation should be obtained before a detailed examination is carried out. However, should such a person not be immediately available, the house surgeon's responsibilities lie with the patient whom he must treat. The police are responsible for the collection of evidence and will ordinarily provide their own doctor who is specially trained in forensic medicine. The police may require the clothing for forensic examination because it may be important evidence. If it has to be removed in a hurry, the house surgeon should ensure that it is taken off with as little damage as possible and that all stains, either wet or dry, and foreign substances such as mud, grass or dust that are on it are preserved. The clothing is put in a clean paper or plastic bag for scientific examination.

Physical examination of the assaulted person should include measurements of his height and weight which are of considerable practicality in assault between men in violent fighting. The following points should be sought and recorded:

1. The situation, number and type of wounds.
2. The size, shape, depth and direction of the wounds.
3. The condition at the edges, the ends and the base.
4. Any foreign bodies attached or embedded in the wounds.
5. Observations on haemorrhage, its source and volume.

In addition to these observations, routine observations of vital signs, particularly of the cardiovascular system, pulse, blood pressure, heart sounds, respiratory rate, and of the central nervous system, level of consciousness, should be made.

It is worth recording these findings in great detail and making clear, simple diagrams and measurements of all wounds. Blood for alcohol levels or drugs should be obtained if there is any suggestion of alcohol or drug abuse. Photography is very valuable in cases of wounding; it is not simply to save making accurate notes but rather to amplify them and to provide refreshment to one's memory when evidence about the incident is required. Photographs have an evidential value of their own, provided safeguards are taken in their developing and printing. Many A and E departments nowadays have Polaroid cameras which will allow quick shots of the wounds to be taken. If the A and E department staff are doing this themselves they are well advised always to stick an adhesive metal tape with the name of the patient and the date on to the patient before the photograph is taken. In many cases of wounding, the police will wish to take their own photographs. This is not of direct concern to the house surgeon, provided it does not in any way compromise the clinical care of the patient. However, the police must obtain the patient's consent before the collection of any photographs or blood samples.

RAPE AND SEXUAL ASSAULT

It must be stressed that the victim of sexual assault is a patient first and foremost and must be treated as such.

If a female alleges a heterosexual assault it is best to assume at the beginning of the interview that rape *has* been committed. Females may present at hospital initially with minor stories of abdominal pain, trivial injuries or bruising and, after admission may allege that they have been the subject of a sexual assault. Ordinarily, such allegations should alert the nursing and medical staff who then report the matter to the police, who will produce their own medical expert to examine the patient. In many cities there are also special centres for victims of rape or sexual assault. The house surgeon may be caught out if he or she has already started to examine a patient who in the course of examination says that they have been the victim of a sexual assault. In these circumstances, the house surgeon is best advised to desist from further examination and to take every possible step to ensure the patient's situation is not altered until a more adequate medical examination can be carried out by an expert. In particular, the nurses should not be allowed to wash or shower such a patient and all clothing from the patient should be carefully collected together and stored in brown paper or plastic bags.

Victims of sexual assault or patients who allege sexual assault deserve considerable sympathy and understanding from the medical and nursing staff. They may have already been subjected to a horrifying intrusion into their privacy and the further examinations that are necessary for the legal process are no less harassing. Useful help in this crisis can be obtained in the UK from voluntary Victims Support Schemes who can send a counsellor to the victim (National Association of Victims Support Schemes, London SW9—Tel. 01-737 2010).

Sexual assault may result in serious injury requiring urgent surgical intervention, for instance a vaginal rupture. In these circumstances it is useful for the operating team to be aware of the requirements of evidence for the courts. These should include pubic hair combings (all the pubic hair should be saved in a clean dry container if the patient is to be shaved prior to surgery), swabs from any bite marks, an introital swab, a perineal swab and a high vaginal swab (which should be obtained after insertion of a sterile unlubricated speculum *before* any internal examination). In cases where buggery is alleged, rectal swabs are indicated. Saliva for secretor status and blood for group, alcohol and drugs are additional investigations.

Appendix I

ENZYME NOMENCLATURE

(Based on the recommendation of the International Union of Biochemistry.)

Official Name (other names or abbreviations in brackets)	Abbreviation
Acid phosphatase	ACP
Alkaline phosphatase	ALP
Amylase (diastase)	AMS
Aspartate transaminase	AST (AAT, SGOT)
Cholinesterase	CHS
Creatine kinase	CK
Lactate dehydrogenase	LD (LDH)
Lipase	LPS
Pepsin	PPS
Trypsin	TPS

Appendix II

SI SYSTEM

The SI (for Système International) unit system now dominates measurement in many countries. Below are the basic SI units with their proper abbreviations and also some of the derived units. Conversion factors are included.

Basic SI units and abbreviations

Length	metre	m
Mass	kilogram	kg
Time	second	s
Electric current	ampere	A
Thermodynamic temperature	kelvin	K
Luminous intensity	candela	cd
Amount of substance	mole	mol

Some derived SI units, abbreviations and definitions

Energy	joule (J)	$kg\ m^2 s^{-2}$
Force	newton (N)	$kg\ m\ s^{-2} = J\ m^{-1}$
Power	watt (W)	$kg\ m^2 s^{-3} = J\ s^{-1}$
Pressure	pascal (Pa)	$kg\ m^{-1}\ s^{-2} = N\ m^{-2}$
Electric charge	coulomb (C)	$A\ s$
Electric potential difference	volt (V)	$kg\ m^2\ s^{-3}\ A^{-1}$ $= J\ A^{-1}\ s^{-1}$
Electric resistance	ohm (Ω)	$kg\ m^2\ s^{-3}\ A^{-2}$ $= V\ A^{-1}$
Electric conductance	siemens (S)	$kg^{-1}\ m^{-2}\ s^3\ A^2$ $= \Omega^{-1}$
Electric capacitance	farad (F)	$A^2\ s^4\ kg^{-1}\ m^{-2}$ $= A\ s\ V^{-1}$
Frequency	hertz (Hz)	s^{-1}
Area	square metre	m^2
Volume	cubic metre	m^3
Velocity	metre per second	$m\ s^{-1}$
Molality	mole per kilogram	$mol\ kg^{-1}$
Concentration	mole per cubic decimetre	$mol\ dm^{-3}$

Prefixes for SI units

Fraction	Prefix	Symbol	Multiple	Prefix	Symbol
10^{-1}	deci	d	10	deca	da
10^{-2}	centi	c	10^2	hecto	h
10^{-3}	milli	m	10^3	kilo	k
10^{-6}	micro	μ	10^6	mega	M
10^{-9}	nano	n	10^9	giga	G
10^{-12}	pico	p	10^{12}	tera	T
10^{-15}	femto	f			
10^{-18}	atto	a			

Interconversions from selected 'old' units to SI units

'Old unit'	Multiplication factor, 'old' to 'new'	SI unit
Calorie (kcal)	4.18	kiloJoule (kJ)
Pressure (mmHg)	0.133	kiloPascal (kPa)
(torr)	0.133	kiloPascal (kPa)
(cmH_2O)	0.098	kiloPascal (kPa)
Radiation (rad)	0.01	Gray (Gy)
(roentgen)	2.58×10^{-4}	Coulomb/kg (C/kg)

Appendix III

LABORATORY REFERENCE RANGES

In most instances the reference ranges given have been obtained from the Institute of Medical and Veterinary Science, South Australia. Where possible, the data conform with the SI system of units.

Haematology

Packed cell volume (PCV, haematocrit)	
Male	0.42–0.52
Female	0.37–0.47
Haemoglobin	
Male	2.09–2.79 mmol/l
Female	1.78–2.56 mmol/l
Erythrocytes	
Male	4.6–6.2×10^9/l
Female	4.2–5.4×10^9/l
Reticulocytes	0.1–4.0%
Mean corpuscular volume (MCV)	80–96 fl
Mean corpuscular haemoglobin (MCH)	0.42–0.48 fmol

Mean corpuscular haemoglobin
   concentration (MCHC)   0.30–0.34
Sedimentation rate
   (ESR)—Westergren
     Male < 5 mm/h
     Female < 7 mm/h
Platelets $150–350 \times 10^9/l$
Leucocytes
   total $4.0–10.0 \times 10^9/l$
   neutrophils $2.5–7.5 \times 10^9/l$
   lymphocytes $1.5–3.5 \times 10^9/l$
   monocytes $200–800 \times 10^9/l$
   eosinophils $40–440 \times 10^9/l$
   plasma cells   occasional
   blast cells   nil
   promyelocytes   nil
   myelocytes   nil
Bleeding time   0.18–0.36 ks
Clotting time   0.24–0.60 ks
Prothrombin time (one stage)   10–12 s
Prothrombin activity   70–100%
Activated partial thromboplastin
   time   30–40 s
Thromboplastin screening test
   (Hicks-Pitney)   8–10 s
Plasma fibrinogen   1.5–4.0 g/l
                           $(0.5–1.3\ \mu mol/l)$
Euglobulin clot lysis time   7.2–18 ks
Serum fibrin degradation products
   (fibrin related antigen)   0–10 mg/l
Serum iron
    Male $8–35\ \mu mol/l$
    Female $8–27\ \mu mol/l$
Serum folate $3–20\ \mu g/l$
Serum vitamin B_{12} 180–1000 pmol/l

Clinical Chemistry—Venous Plasma Concentrations

Sodium	137–145 mmol/l
Potassium	3.1–4.2 mmol/l
Calcium	2.2–2.6 mmol/l
Magnesium	0.7–0.9 mmol/l
Copper	
males	10–22 μmol/l
females	10–30 μmol/l
females on oral contraceptives	15–35 μmol/l
Iron	12–32 μmol/l
Zinc	9–19 μmol/l
Chloride	98–106 mmol/l
Bicarbonate	22–32 mmol/l
Phosphate	0.7–1.3 mmol/l
Lactate	0.7–1.8 mmol/l
Pyruvate	0.06–0.12 mmol/l
Urea	3–8 mmol/l
Creatinine	50–120 μmol/l
Uric acid	150–450 μmol/l
Glucose (fasting)	3.8–5.8 mmol/l
Cholesterol	4–8 mmol/l
Triglyceride	0.3–2.0 mmol/l
Bilirubin	6–24 μmol/l
Protein	
total	65–81 g/l
albumin	34–45 g/l
transferrin	2.0–4.0 g/l
immunoglobulin G	8.0–16.0 g/l
immunoglobulin A	1.6–4.0 g/l
immunoglobulin M	0.8–2.0 g/l
fibrinogen	1.5–4.0 g/l
Osmolality	285–290 mosmol/kg
Ammonia	<50 μmol/l

Clinical Chemistry—Arterial Blood or Plasma

pH	7.38–7.42 pH units
Hydrogen ion activity (H^+)	38–42 nmol/l
Plasma bicarbonate	22–31 mmol/l
CO_2 tension (P_aCO_2)	35–45 mmHg (4.7–6.0 kPa)
O_2 tension (P_aO_2)	75–100 mmHg (10–13.3 kPa)

Clinical Chemistry—Plasma Clearance Values

Bromsulphthalein retention	<0.05 in 45 minutes
Creatinine clearance	
Male	75–190 ml/minute
Female	85–160 ml/minute

Clinical Chemistry—Serum Enzymes

Acid phosphatase (ACP)	2.3–5.7 U/l
Alkaline phosphatase (ALP)	30–110 U/l
Amylase (AMS)	70–300 U/l
Aspartate Transaminase (AST)	10–45 U/l
Lactate dehydrogenase (LDS)	110–230 U/l
Pseudocholinesterase	4–12 U/ml
Creatinine kinase (CK)	
Male	80–360 U/l
Female	40–180 U/l

Clinical Chemistry—24-hour Urine Excretion

Sodium	30–300 mmol
Potassium	30–150 mmol
Calcium (normal diet)	2.5–7.5 mmol
Chloride	30–300 mmol
Phosphate	13–55 mmol
Urea	1.7–5.9 μmol
Urobilinogen	< 70 μmol

Catecholamines	
total	100–600 nmol
noradrenaline	10–300 nmol
adrenaline	10–300 nmol
5-HIAA	< 50 μmol
Hydroxyproline	< 300 μmol
Amylase	200–1000 U

Clinical Chemistry—72-hour Faeces

Fat	< 18 g

Index

INDEX